A Viral Maze

Bertha Amarni

ISBN: 9781511699754

ISBN-13: 9781511699754

Printed by CreateSpace, Charleston SC

In memory of Jane,

because you understood without knowing.

Contents

A Viral Maze

"As you set out for Ithaka hope the voyage is a long one, full of adventure, full of discovery. Laistrygonians and Cyclops, angry Poseidon, don't fear them…" –

Constantine P. Cavafy, 1911

Preface

When I set out on my journey to Ithaka, it was bound to be a wild adventure, for I had a hitchhiker strapped to my back, though little did I know it. Barely a decade after I was officially diagnosed with the hepatitis B virus (HBV), the terrain has improved immensely for those who discover for the first time that they are afflicted by this rather crafty, resilient but silent virus. Then, my life was thrown into confusion. It was a daily grind looking for answers to my most basic questions about how the virus would be likely to affect my life even more than it had already done, how to best manage my day-to-day existence and how to plan for the future. These are not matters you chat to the medical professionals about. Even learning the basic science to enable me understands my blood test results was a struggle.

Since early childhood I had experienced a number of seemingly unconnected chronic illnesses, and I had known intuitively that there was an underlying, undiagnosed problem with my health. Nonetheless, I was still thrown into a state of shock by the diagnosis of chronic active hepatitis B. For months afterwards, I functioned at the level of a robot. First, there was a period of mourning. Then anger. Then fear. Fear of the unknown. I began to panic. I went into hibernation both socially and professionally. I adopted a low impact life, as though that would conserve my energy and prolong my now, as I saw it, blighted life. It took me years to arrive at the equilibrium that has helped me begin to thrive again. I was therefore thrilled some years after I was first diagnosed to discover William Finley Green's brilliant and thoughtful book Hepatitis B: The First Year, published in 2002. The book is a guide for the newly diagnosed to help navigate the conundrum of medical care, daily survival issues and overall mental and emotional health. There have been other important books on living with HBV during the past decade. However, William Finley Green's book has a particular resonance for me, coming from a "patient-expert". If you are newly diagnosed, it tells you all you need to know to understand the medical terminology and blood test results. It gives you an overview of common symptoms and how you might deal with them, where to find information and how to approach finding a good specialist, the current state of therapies and much, much more. I salute him for an extraordinary achievement. Even for a veteran-patient such as I am, I see his book as an essential source to which I will refer again and again as I continue to strive to thrive.

This book is a different type of book. It is a very personal account of my own convoluted journey from seemingly unconnected chronic conditions manifesting from infancy, over more than four decades, to the eventual diagnosis of chronic HBV. My experience shows how the HBV virus can silently spin a spider's web of other chronic conditions while going completely undetected. But above all, it is a story of resilience and survival, of the HBV virus as much of its human host. It is our good fortune that being diagnosed with chronic HBV, even where the virus leads to a myriad other conditions, is no longer a death sentence. You can take charge of your health and still thrive!

Chapter One

Introduction: A Wellness Freak

In Greek mythology, Nemesis noticed the pride and disdains of Narcissus, the son of the river god Cephisus, and attracted him to a pool. Narcissus fell in love with his own reflection in the water and, unable to leave the beauty of his reflection, he shriveled and died. Fixation with oneself can manifest in many different ways. It does not have to be explicitly admiring or overbearing, as it was in the myth of Narcissus. In my case it has been an obsession with my illusive, chronic ill health throughout most of my life and my determination to defeat it. While determination may in itself be a good thing, I did not always know what the culprit was, I did not have a plan, I lacked discipline and, ironically, the absence of a reflecting mirror led me to years of excessive research on anything that could have a positive or negative impact on my health. I would then follow up with spending substantial amounts of money visiting complementary health care professionals, nutritional supplements and physical therapies. I became a wellness freak. All the while I was also seeing physicians who seemed at times as puzzled by my symptoms as I was.

Over time I became accustomed to suffering alone and in silence. Although I did not live alone, the busy lives of family members meant that I shared only the barest facts of my various conditions with them. Young people need to look forward to their own futures without the burden of the nearly spent lives of their parents. Would they have the time to help me with research or accompany me on medical appointments? Would they be truly interested in the information I gathered and tried to incorporate into my life, or would they recoil from my emphasis on naturopathic approaches and especially nutritional healing and whole foods? Would they share good-natured jokes about me and my extreme intolerance of smoke-filled rooms and certain smells that made me feel ill, causing me to flee from restaurants and thus embarrassing them in front of family and friends? A varied range of reactions did manifest, although there was also deep love and compassion between us. Ultimately I began to feel I was on my own. Feeling alone led to states of confusion and terror. On the one hand I knew my family loved me. On the other hand they didn't seem to get it. Long episodes of depression followed, which I only now recognize as depression. I mourned for the very promising professional life that I had developed and which now seemed to begin to falter. I took several long breaks from work. I could do so only because I was a partner in the business. But I was also accountable to colleagues. Poverty beckoned, but not wanting to be seen as a hopeless hypochondriac, I did not speak about my health problems with my partners. No, especially when I did not have a clear understanding of what they were. One diagnosis after another however, things began to become clearer. First, acute mitral valve prolapse, then rheumatoid arthritis, followed by the inflammatory eye disease known as uveitis or iritis, and eventually HBV. In what order did they actually afflict me?

The HBV virus spins an intricate web of chronic conditions. Liver specialists focus on the liver, in the same way that heart specialists focus on the heart or the ophthalmologists on the eyes and, to the detriment of the patient and to the detriment of medical science, the twain often never do meet. Yet although HBV is a liver disease, the first manifestations of the virus may emerge elsewhere in the body. The liver, the largest glandular organ in the body, performs multiple functions that are critical to ridding the entire body of toxins and harmful substances. The fragmented approach of medical practice and patient care means that necessary systemic investigations are not made and the agony of not knowing what you have can drag on for years and years and years. Those of us who have the HBV virus may first experience it in many different ways not obviously linked to the liver. My own experience bears this out. My search for a diagnosis and a sense of resolution spanned more than two decades of my adult life, quite apart from my range of childhood illnesses. A lot happened during that time. Now at last, I have knowledge and medical specialists who I trust, who have helped me manage the conditions reasonably well. I have come to understand the constant fatigue, the brain fog, the migraine headaches, mood swings, palpitations and breathlessness. I understand how they may all relate to each other. I also know how to manage or ameliorate them. I have arrived at a place of calm. I know I have chronic Hepatitis B (HBV), acute mitral valve prolapse, uveitis (an eye inflammation) and joint inflammation. I have at last been able to exhale and get on with life. But the discovery and naming of these health conditions were far from straight forward. It has been the life of a sleuth, and the detective work still goes on in a sense. And in my 'whodunit' assessment of all these health conditions, HBV seems to be the clear culprit.

Global statistics on HBV and other viral liver diseases and morbidity spell disaster for the future. The institution by the World Health Organization of a World Hepatitis Day on 28th July every year to increase awareness and understanding of viral hepatitis bears witness to this reality. According to the WHO, more than 240 million people worldwide have chronic viral hepatitis, and close to a million people die every year as a result of hepatitis B. In HBV endemic regions of the world, infants and children bear the brunt of this destructive viral disease. This is because 90% of them are unable to overcome the acute form of the infection due to their weaker immune defense. Thus, in infants and young children, acute viral infection from which 95% of adults make a full recovery tends to take root, becoming chronic HBV for which there is as yet no definitive cure. In highly endemic regions of the world, the virus is commonly transmitted from mother to child at birth or from child to child during early childhood. Mother to child transmission is said to also account for more than 30% of chronic infections in low endemic regions. No other member of my family, including my now very elderly parents, has been found to have HBV or has suffered with chronic ill health the way I have. Baby boomers have different stories to tell. For a few of us, illness has been a lifelong companion. But many have been far luckier and may only experience chronic illness in their twilight years. My story is one that I want to share. If you are living with a chronic condition, or two, or three, or indeed four as I am, it helps to hear other stories. Be they happier or sadder than your own, they can offer insights or comfort. And if you are one of the lucky ones, it helps to count your blessings. If you are still young and are experiencing niggling episodes of ill health, and especially if you live in HBV prone regions such as China, South East Asia, Africa, even in the United States and Eastern Europe, I urge you to get tested and get advice about possible vaccination against HBV. Surely prevention is better than a non-existent cure?

I am constantly amazed at what a dance life can still be in the midst of illness or misfortune. Many years ago I came across and was deeply touched by Constantine Cavafy 's beautiful epic poem 'Ithaka' and adopted it as my companion poem. Cavafy was born in 1863 in Alexandria, Egypt, to Greek parents, and was baptized into the Greek Orthodox Church. His father had lived in England prior to his birth and had British nationality. During a period of war and social strife in Alexandria, Cavafy took his family to live in Liverpool, England, but returned to Alexandria when peace returned. He experienced other episodes of exile from

Bertha Amarni

Alexandria due to war and social and political disturbance, forcing him to travel widely, but always returning to the city of Alexandria. His poems were published in the form of broadsheets for his friends and only gained public recognition toward the end of his life. The poem Ithaka has special resonance. And so wise! It helps restore a swing to the step when the spirit begins to sag and it has helped me remain philosophical in embracing my life in spite of the challenges. Now a famous poem, Ithaka has gained cult status among some college students. If you are not familiar with the poem, I urge you to read and meditate upon it.

Chapter Two

In Sync with Hepatitis B?

Yesterday I went to see my Hepatologist in a large city hospital. I shall call him Dr H. Dr H reviewed my latest blood tests and liver ultrasound results with me. I have lost count of how many times I have visited his consulting suite. I used to see him four times a year when my viral load was in the stratosphere. But for quite a few years now I have seen him just twice a year. These appointments, and other regular medical appointments have become fixtures in my diary. For the past few years my test results have been so consistently good that Dr H once suggested that I might save myself the trouble of making the regular visits to see him and resort to a telephone consultation instead. I smiled and thanked him for his consideration. But I told him these visits have become an important part of my year. I actually look forward to them. Sometimes they are very short because the virus has been undetectable for a long while. At other times I have lots of questions for him. Questions he is always willing to answer in the most direct way. He does not hesitate to say 'I'm afraid I don't know the answer' or 'well, I haven't heard that before'. When he asks about my health, my professional life or what book I am reading, he seems genuinely interested. If I ask for a copy of the blood test results, he walks me to the nurses' room and requests a copy for me, spreading his calm and brightness along the corridor. Someone did a terrific job raising this very cultured man. On top of it all, he is quite a looker! No sir, thank you very much but I do not want a telephone consultation. You reassure and cheer me up! Talking to you down the telephone line can never be the same. The eye contact that tells me it's alright to press and challenge what he tells me, the care he takes to explain the blood test results as he scrolls down the screen to show me. I am a fan.

Yesterday's consultation was unremarkable in its outcome. My last liver function tests were normal and my viral load still undetectable. My most recent ultrasound showed "no complications of the liver disease". I asked about the two small cysts on my kidney that the radiologist had mentioned at the time of my scan. It turns out a much earlier test had recorded it as well. Dr H tells me my kidney markers are fine and that 20% of perfectly healthy people have kidney cysts. He will keep an eye on it. I tell him I would like a review of my liver fibrosis status as it is now some six years since my liver biopsy. He will arrange for me to have a fibroscan, a newer, non-invasive fibrosis test, in time for my next visit. My current prescription for the drug Entecavir was continued. As for the blood tes results, Dr H said he couldn't be happier. As before, all markers are within normal ranges and in particular the virus is 'completely undetectable', with my liver function tests 'entirely normal'. I still ask him the question that I always ask. How infectious am I? 'You are not infectious, you are no more infectious than I am', he tells me. We agree on another review in six months and I stride out of his consulting room with a smile on my face and a spring in my step. But mind you, visits to hepatologists were not always such a wholesome experience. I have been around the block a few times, trying to find a specialist who struck just the right tone. One very lovely patrician had put me on a drug with which I disagreed for a number of reasons. So my physician referred me to Dr H for a second opinion. He agreed with my assessment of the risks of serious side effects. He offered me Entecavir and an excellent working relationship and I have never looked back.

Bertha Amarni

When I was officially diagnosed with HBV more than a decade or so ago, I had been in limbo for quite a few years. I had suspected for some time that there might be something wrong with my liver. The immediate event that led to the diagnosis was the result of a blood test done in the course of a medical examination for a prospective employer. To this day I am eternally grateful for the circumstances that brought me to that point. The physician who performed the examination had identified other health issues that I already knew about, and he seemed surprised that I had highly elevated liver enzymes. He asked if I knew why, and I told him I didn't but that I had suspected there was a problem and told him why. He suggested I see my general physician for a liver test as soon as possible, which I proceeded to do. As for the job for which the medical was conducted, I was appointed to the post and did hold it for a few years. However, it was a very demanding senior position involving a considerable amount of foreign travel. I eventually resigned from it because I was constantly exhausted and was diagnosed with chronic fatigue. The first liver test ordered by my physician was positive for HBV. However, I had received a first dose of the HBV vaccine the week before the medical examination that first noted my elevated liver enzymes. My doctor reasonably thought that the vaccine might have affected the test results. He therefore asked me to repeat the test six months later.

A Viral Maze

The second test result was definitively positive for HBV, confirming an intermediate test I had had when I felt poorly while on a business trip. The technician who handed the results to me at the clinic then wore the solemn face of an undertaker. Expecting me to become emotional, he stared at me with sadness in his eyes. He asked if I wanted some water or a cup of coffee.

Back home six months after my very first blood test and with that result now confirmed by a second, my physician and I agreed that I should find a specialist to look after me. We discussed two hepatologists he recommended. I was concerned I had not been given the choice of a woman. Nonetheless I selected one of the two and a referral was made. My first visit to the consulting rooms of my first hepatologist was fairly routine. My viral load was apparently moderate, according to my blood test results. He thought the virus was unlikely to have affected my DNA. On our second consultation however, he said I should undergo a second test to resolve that question. When I did, the results were disappointingly positive. The virus had affected my DNA. I sat across the desk from the hepatologist when he gave me the news, with words including 'unfortunately'. I made no response for some considerable time. When I eventually spoke, it was to ask if the results could indicate how long I had had the virus. I of course wanted to find out how I might have contracted the disease. I was concerned about contagion and how to protect my loved ones and ensure that I have not and do not pass it on to others with whom I come into contact. He made some comment about my not being under any obligation to spread the word outside my immediate family. I understood that, but I had no concern whatever at the time if the whole world knew that I have the HBV virus. Then there was a sudden rush of blood to my head and a tingling down my spine. I felt a sense of elation. At last it was conclusive. My malaise had a name. I had chronic, active HBV. My viral load was high enough and other relevant markers raised concern. But the mystery was solved, at last! I left the consulting room feeling vindicated after many years of searching for the reason I was always tired, sometimes emotional, easily upset, occasionally fainted and often generally unwell. I was often hardly ill enough to say I was ill, but on the other hand hardly well enough to wake up in the morning feeling bright and energetic and revving to go. Of course I wanted my world to know. I had not been losing my mind.

When I got home I made phone calls to my family and friends. They needed to know that I do have the silent killer HBV! But soon exhilaration turned into anger, then fear and eventually withdrawal. Why the anger? I had always known what a lottery life can be, and I am not the worst victim of cosmic randomness. I had been spared the randomness of being born into abject poverty or famine or in the midst of war. But being philosophical in accepting my situation still did not assuage my need to know just how I had picked up the virus and when.

I have lived a rather chaste life for a baby boomer who entered college on the West Coast in the mid-seventies. I never tried weed and definitely did not inject myself with anything, medicinal or recreational. I didn't smoke or drink. I was in my early twenties when I married my first sexual partner who is still in very good health and does not have HBV. I proceeded to have three children in my twenties and tried to pursue a very challenging professional career along with raising my children. However I have, for as far back as I can remember, had a pervasive sense that there was something fundamentally the matter with my health. This suspicion was based on the many episodes of illness during my early childhood most of which I still vividly remember as if I am watching a film screen and a few of which have become part of the family lore. The sleuth in me stirred. I have to go back to the beginning and piece it all together. I have to follow the scent. But this would come later. After sending out an alert to what I call my at risk network, I asked each member of my family to attend a physician to have a blood test. My stubborn husband resisted the request for many weeks but eventually relented and was tested. My children were more mature about it and went together to have the test done. My entire family was found to be free of the virus and they proceeded to receive the vaccine. I much later realized that the question whether or not they had an immunity to the virus should have been specifically addressed before they were given the vaccine. But this was not. The one question that might have helped me establish how long I had had the virus had not been answered. An attempt to retrace the steps failed to yield any helpful information. And in any event, I recalled that my own diagnosis had been inconclusive for more than six months precisely because I had not been tested for the virus before being given a dose of the vaccine. If, as HBV specialists have told me an infected mother does not necessarily pass on the virus to her baby, then my family and I have had an amazing good luck in the midst of what I regard to be a tragedy. It is also true that my childbirth years have been the healthiest I have ever known, my youngest having been born when I was 28. This may well have coincided with a dormant period of the virus which can apparently alternate between long periods of dormancy and activity.

Months of melancholy followed as I tried to make sense of all the information, there were months of melancholy. And then a furious pace of research about everything that could possibly impact my new found HBV status. I spent weeks on nutrition and supplements. I consulted a conventional physician who is also a nutritionist. I seemed to think I could overcome the virus without resorting to pharmaceuticals. I resorted to massage, acupuncture and yoga and got myself a gym membership. I spent my savings on whole foods and exotic superfoods and physical therapies. They kept me healthy and surprisingly energetic. And for a while my viral load, initially moderately high, seemed to decrease. But that seeming improvement was short lived.

Chapter Three

Fear of Sunlight, and the Chinese Perspective

I was on holiday with my brother in a sunny beach town. We rented a house near the water, expecting our respective families to join us for a few days. I woke up from what seemed a good night's sleep. I could only tell it was broad daylight because of the intensity of birdsong around me and the rays of the sun on my face. I remained on by back in bed. I thought how odd it was that my head felt so heavy. I was aware that in spite of the birdsong and the feel of the sun's rays on my face, it was still dark. I lay in darkness and my head was beginning to throb. I tried to open my eyes. I could not. It seemed as if a strong force of gravity was holding the lids down and any attempt to resist it was met with excruciating pain. I made several attempts to tweak one eyelid open, but in vain, I let out a plaintive cry that brought my brother hurrying into my room. He helped me up and into the bathroom and stayed with me as I tried and failed to open my eyes, and then tried again. I eventually managed to open one eye and then the other. I looked up into the bathroom mirror. One of my eyes was completely blood shot, the other quite pink, and tears streamed down my face. It was a Sunday and shops and pharmacies were closed. Thinking that it might be an eye infection, perhaps a severe form of conjunctivitis, my brother fetched warm salty water in a glass and persuades me to bathe my eyes with it. I did so as well as I could. My eyes stung badly from the salt water. But that was nothing compared with the pain I felt in both eyes from the bright daylight. I spent the rest of the morning indoors with my dark glasses on and my eyes half closed most of the time. By evening, I felt a bit better and we moved around the house by candlelight. I was deeply shaken by the experience, and so was my brother. I remember telling him that the pain I felt was more excruciating and frightening than any thing I had felt before. It was in a league of its own. Much, much worse than labor pains, of which I had ample experience.

That morning was the beginning of five years of physical and emotional agony which ended in having the lenses in both my eyes replaced in two cataract operations. The complications that followed one of the operations are still not completely resolved so many years later. I returned home from the beach the next day and went to the emergency clinic of my local general hospital. I was referred to an ophthalmologist I shall refer to as Dr O, under whose care I remained for many years. Uveitis was diagnosed without any hesitation whatsoever. I was prescribed an eye drop called Maxidex. The Belgian pharmaceutical company Alcon-Couvreur manufactures Maxidex. Among other things, the drug contains dexamethasone, a corticosteroid. It is often used to reduce inflammation following eye surgery and is to be phased out as quickly as possible given its tendency to cause a build up of pressure in the eye that can lead to glaucoma, cataracts, and other nasty possible side effects. Dr O advised that I remain on the Maxidex for one week and then begin phasing it out by reducing the dose from one drop four times a day to three times, then two, then one, at intervals of three days until I stopped using it completely.

Uveitis, also known as iritis, is an inflammation of the uvea of the eye. It is said to have many causes including autoimmune disease, viral infection and trauma. Some are idiopathic, meaning the cause is unknown. The condition makes the eyes ultra sensitive to light of any kind, but especially bright sunlight. It causes excriciating pain. In investigating what might have caused the condition in me, Dr O asked whether I had experienced any physical trauma or had rheumatoid arthritis that may have led to the eye inflammation. I did have some joint pain that seemed to flare up periodically and then subside. This had been going on for many years, prompting me to see a Rheumatologist who did not think my rheumatoid factor gave cause for concern. Initially it registered a low reading and then seemed to disappear. I was never asked about infections, nor was my liver ever mentioned. However, without the benefit of internet research I recalled a common claim that there is a link between the liver and the eye. Perhaps it is just one of those gems from folk wisdom which one picks up while growing up, and I kept thinking about it. I also thought of the jaundiced eyes of a janitor I knew who died from advanced liver disease. Although my eyes were not jaundiced, the link between the liver and the eyes was not in doubt. I did some library research, although much of what I found was either too basic, or in very technical medical books I found difficult to comprehend. I eventually found a small paperback in a health food store devoted to the liver, but it contained nothing that made me any wiser about my uveitis. At this early stage I was fully expecting my uveitis to clear up fairly quickly. I was not that troubled by the use of the Maxidex drops. I decided to focus on being as well as I could possibly be in all other respects. It was at this time that I decided to consult a doctor at a highly recommended traditional Chinese medical practice.

I was primarily in search of some therapy to help me relax and boost my energy level. I saw a charming lady Physician who is an orthodox MD as well as qualified in Chinese traditional medicine. I told her I wanted to ensure that my general health was in peak condition. I made regular weekly visits for acupuncture and massage and green teas, and she checked my pulse and listened to my heart. I had kept these visits up for more than a year when she checked my pulse one day and looked at me quizzically. As she held my wrist in her hand she said, 'your liver blood is weak. We have to watch it'. I asked her to explain her meaning and she said it meant my liver function was not good enough. She told me to go to my general physician and ask for a liver function test. I did so. My physician said my blood test results were normal and gave no cause for concern. My Chinese doctor seemed unimpressed with my physician's finding. She went as far as saying she thought my liver was implicated in my eye inflammation. After a few more of my regular weekly visits, she told me that the weakness in my liver blood was getting more pronounced and I should go back to my physician and ask for screening for liver disease. I did so. My Physician seemed somewhat bemused, but ordered another blood test, which came back negative for whatever liver disease he tested for. At this point I had very little knowledge of hepatitis of any kind, and I cannot tell you precisely what tests were performed. However, I remember my physician telling me that my lifestyle did not raise any concerns for liver disease. I also remember thinking, how could he possibly know where I have been and what I have been exposed to? However, I appreciated that he meant well by that comment, even if it was misguided. At a loss about what to do, I consulted a naturopathic doctor highly recommended by a friend. She advised me to undergo a liver cleanse and referred me to colleagues who specialized in this from a rather posh address at exorbitant fees. It was a weeklong program that included some fasting, drinking of various vegetable juices and an enema. What I felt at the end of it was emotional exhaustion and not in the least bit physically energized. It was shortly after this liver detoxification that a routine job related medical examination found my liver enzymes to be abnormally high. I asked for a copy of the blood test results for my own doctor. After two further blood tests ordered by mygeneral physician, as previously mentioned, I was confirmed to have the HBV virus, in its chronic active form.

Why did my Chinese Doctor persist in trying to establish that my eye problem was connected to my liver function when my orthodox doctors did not explore that connection at all, and in fact no other possible connection seriously? Be they generalists or specialists, these doctors were good enough doctors. What made them so disinclined to dig deeper and make what must sometimes be glaring connections to the trained professional eye? Furthermore, the role of viral infection in causing inflammation in the body generally and of the eye is, I now know, frequently referred to in medical information now easily available on the worldwide web. Although the warnings accompanying the Maxidex eye drops highlighted the risk of cataracts if used for extended periods of time and warned against prolonged use, my eyes seemed to develop what can only be called an addiction to the drug. After the first two weeks of use, in accordance with my doctor's advice I slowly tapered use and came off altogether. Both eyes were quiet for nearly two weeks. Then the inflammation flared up with a vengeance. I was placed back on the drops and from then onwards, for nearly five years, the longest period I was off the drops was about eleven weeks, before I had a flare up. I was tempted to abandon the drug completely and damn the consequences. I thought if I went cold turkey I could face whatever flare-ups and withdrawal symptoms followed. But I was warned against that. The ophthalmologist I was then seeing told me the alternative to not using the drops may be too horrific to contemplate. I could loose my sight. I was terrified. I started researching for natural alternatives, but the Internet did not at that time offer anywhere as much information as it does now. What I did find was a Russian plant extract for clearing cataracts. I ordered several bottles from a source in Cyprus and even telephoned to discuss my condition and the medication with the chemist proprietor. In the end, I did not feel I knew enough about it or any possible side effects and did not use it.

After a year or so of the stops and starts with Maxidex eye drops, my rather high-pressured professional life had been badly affected. I needed to take stock of my situation and develop a plan B in the event that I could no longer continue with my current position and needed to modify or drastically change the way I worked. I reflected with trusted friends. One such friend told me of a former colleague of hers who had suffered from the condition and might be able to talk me through some of the hoops she had to navigate and the aids and gadgets and health insurance benefits that might be available. She put us in touch, and although we never met, we spent time on the phone and I gained an awful lot from her generosity in sharing her rather painful experience with such good humor. This lady had been on Maxidex eye drops for a whole year, trying and failing to successfully wean herself off it. Her body then reacted violently to the steroid and she literally swelled up. In the end she got fed up with it all and stopped using the drops. Her weight slowly returned to normal. But she lost the sight in both of her eyes. What I learned from her, convinced me that if I were to lose my sight, I would want to be well prepared to be able to continue my professional life as seamlessly as possible. And it set me on a journey that began with consultations with an Association for the Visually Impaired. There I was offered some counseling and was given a tour of a range of gadgets to help with dictating and typing. I was particularly impressed with an app that plugs into your computer and types away as you dictate. I bought it and took it home with me and spent my weekends learning to use it effectively. It really was pretty basic at the time, but I understand that the device has now been considerably upgraded and improved. Although my family understood the logic in my wanting to be prepared just in case, they were rather alarmed to have to even contemplate the possibility. I was still grappling with uveitis and the maxidex eye drops when I was officially diagnosed with the HBV virus – a lag of some three and a half years.

Then one bright and sunny morning another year or so later while still on the maxidex eye drops, I sat at my desk in my office working my way through a file of reports. I use reading glasses normally and I had no difficulty that morning reading with them on. My office was a large room with a conference table seating 12 and bookshelves lining opposite walls of the room. It had a private door that opened onto a terrace, and there was also an adjoining door between my office and the office of my secretary. When you entered my office from the office of the secretary, you would face my desk that stood some 20 feet from the door. There was a faint tap on the interconnecting door. Someone entered the room. When I looked up towards the door, the head of the person was a hazy blob and I could not tell who it was. It was as if a light excluding screen had come down in front of my eyes. Not until he was directly in front of me did I make out whom it was. I concealed my dismay and we completed our discussion. I rose from my desk and paced around the room. I went into the washroom and closed the door. I looked in the mirror but could see no obvious change to the colour or clarity of my pupils. I shut the left eye, which was the eye more aggressively affected by the uveitis. I looked ahead through the right eye. I detected no problem with my vision in that eye. But when I reversed the process and looked through the left eye, my close up vision may have had a bit of a rain cloud feel about it but was not worryingly poor. I returned to my desk and looked across in the distance at a bookshelf near the door. I could not distinguish the books on the shelf one from the other. Something was clearly wrong and it was to do with my distance vision. I walked out on to the terrace and looked across to the trees and benches in a nearby park I was very familiar with. The view was no more than a haze.

I made an emergency appointment with my Ophthalmologist and I went to see him the next morning. He put me through the usual paces of examination. We then returned to his desk in silence. For a few minutes, he continued in silence flipping back through my notes. I found that ominous, as if he was gathering the courage to give me extremely bad news. Should I break the silence and make his job easier? But being an experienced specialist, this would not be his first time having to break bad news to a patient. In my mind I quickly ran through my box file of notes, addresses and the app that I had bought from the Society for the Visually Impaired. How much outstanding leave did I still have from the previous calendar year? I made a mental list of my financial outgoings and was about to tackle my income when he cleared his throat and looked up from the file. You have cataracts in both eyes, he said. It is more advanced in the left eye, he told me. He also told me the backs of both eyes were in good health. I did not reveal my ultimate sense of relief, because I had seen him six weeks previously and was surprised that there had been no sign of cataracts then. I had heard that steroid induced cataracts can be extremely aggressive, but I could not have imagined it could rear its head and advance so quickly within just six weeks. I said so. He said he had noted some months ago that I was developing cataracts. I said I should have been told. He said he mentioned it. I said I was unlikely to forget if he had told me. He said in his Boston practice this exchange would never have happened because he always had an assistant to take down the notes. Be that as it may, we now had to deal with the cataracts. The left eye had become so poor that he thought that should be dealt with straight away. What about continued use of the maxidex eye drops? He repeated his previous advice. It is the only reasonable means available to control my eye inflammation and the risk of not controlling it is more serious than getting cataracts. It was clear to me that I had hardly any choice in the matter now. But I thought I should speak to my family before I made an appointment for surgery. I then sought a second opinion from another ophthalmologist. She confirmed the previous advice. I liked her warmth and directness and the atmosphere in her consulting rooms. I decided to transfer to her and I arranged for the surgery to be done by her. It happened less than a week later. It was under local anesthetic and went very swiftly, without incident. I was in a recovery room for about three hours and was then discharged to go home. We made an appointment for the right eye to be done in eight weeks, if the eye remained quiet of uveitis.

Unfortunately, the condition flared up again when I tried to phase out the drops four weeks after the first operation. So the second operation had to be postponed, in fact there were three postponements, the last because of work travel commitments. It finally took place six months after the first. But six months later, with further maxidex use, the cataract in the right eye had thickened so much that it was not the simple procedure the first one had been. And it was clearly very awkward for the surgeon and her team. Being under local anesthetic, I was fully aware of what was going on, which must have restrained the team from saying too much to each other. In fact I was aware they were being restrained in what they said. Under local anesthetic, I lay on the operating table for well over an hour while the surgeon struggled to remove the lens, necessitating a topping up of the initial dose of anesthetic. When she finally finished, she said 'this hasn't been an easy operation, I am sure you realized that'.

When I was wheeled into the recovery room my daughter who had been waiting was obviously relieved to see me and hurried to inspect me to see, as she joked, if I had accidentally lost a body part. What did go wrong was that my pupil was a bit squashed and has resulted in astigmatism in that eye in which I had previously had almost twenty/twenty vision. And seven years after my cataract operations, the risk of a flare up of the inflammation is never too far from my reality. When two years ago I had to have a laser (YAG) procedure to trim away a thickening of the capsule edges in the left eye, the inflammation flared up again and, with the use of maxidex, took some twelve weeks to subside. The right eye now requires the same procedure and I cannot but hold my breath until the procedure and its almost inevitable accompanying uveitis flare-up is over. Inevitably, it will leave behind the accumulation of even more floaters in both eyes.

Chapter Four

Prolapsed Mitral Valve

In my early thirties, a routine visit to my family doctor, doctor R, left me in shock. It was in the middle of winter and a stubborn cold had done the rounds in my family. When it got to me it was aggressive and was unusually protracted. I went to see doctor R, a kindly middle-aged man who had known my family for many years. I lay on his couch as he listened to my chest with his stethoscope. I saw a sudden rather worried look cross his face. I asked him what he had found that made him look so worried. He said, come and sit down. Back at his desk he said 'you have a heart murmur, a very pronounced heart murmur. I haven't heard one this loud in my entire career. We must get you to the hospital'. Now, my doctor was in his mid-sixties and was planning to retire later that year. As I sat in his patient's chair I could feel and hear my heart pumping very loud. That was not the first time I was hearing it. I had never thought of speaking to anyone about it. I just assumed everyone heard their heart pumping. My doctor suggested calling an ambulance to take me to the hospital. But I had driven myself quite competently to his practice. I was sure it was no emergency and I promised to take myself to see the cardiologist. So I was spared the drama of an ambulance. I was prescribed an antibiotic for the cold and a priority appointment was made for me to see a cardiologist.

I soon received a phone call from the hospital asking me to go in for an echocardiogram (ECG), and an exercise test on a treadmill. After these tests I saw the cardiologist. His diagnosis was that I had a moderately severe prolapsed mitral valve and there was some enlargement of the heart. He saw no need for any intervention at this stage, but I should be reviewed in three months. If things remained stable there would be six-monthly follow-ups after that. Then the prognosis: I wanted to know what the worst-case scenario would be. He told me if replacement of the valve became necessary it would have to be replaced with a pig's skin valve or a mechanical valve. He thought however that it looked perfectly repairable in its current condition. My reaction to that information was very negative. He reassured me I was in no mortal danger as matters stood and could be kept under regular review for the next few years. So we agreed to do just that. There was no need for any drug therapy with the exception that I would need to be given antibiotic before any dental procedure and I should let my dentist know of the condition in advance of attending any appointments. How did this happen to me? He asked if I had had rheumatic fever as an infant. I did not know the answer to that but I knew I had had chronic childhood illnesses that remained undiagnosed, and seemed to resolve after a while. I also know that I had had a prolonged illness after a childhood vaccination. But we shall return to this aspect later in the book.

My prolapsed mitral valve manifested in many different ways during the years that followed. There were periodic chest pains, extreme fatigue, a racing heart, altitude sickness, high blood pressure and finally breathlessness. But it was the altitude sickness that finally got my goat because its consequences for my career were so far reaching. I had competed for and won a senior position with a leading international organization. I served the first year of the appointment in the United States and was transferred to Nairobi for two years in the first instance. The position involved a lot of international travel. While I enjoyed this aspect of the job, I began to notice that every time I returned to Nairobi I had protracted bouts of dizziness and fatigue. And on occasions my eyes were blood shot. Rather than improve over time, this seemed to get more pronounced. Every time I returned from a trip abroad, it seemed that I had to acclimatize to the altitude all over again. I just could not cope with it. I sought transfer to a different station within the organization but there was no vacancy in my field anywhere else. In the end I decided to resign from the position and thus returned to live at sea level once again. The symptoms of altitude sickness disappeared. I have since been back to Nairobi on only one occasion, for a weeklong conference. Within a few days the dizziness and blood shot eyes appeared once again. They disappeared just as quickly once I left. As the years went by the prolapse seemed to stabilize, according to my cardiologist. Although it was apparently getting no worse, it was nonetheless bad enough and my heart had to work harder to maintain effective blood circulation. The enlargement of the heart progressed a little. The tricuspid valve eventually began to leak also, apparently a direct result of the added burden placed on it by an inefficient mitral valve.

By the time I was fifty, my cardiologist was repeatedly advising that it was time to surgically repair both valves. Also worrying was the fact that every time I had an ultrasound of my heart the technicians seemed completely taken aback by how bad the prolapse was and the amount of blood that just flowed out into the void. On one occasion a technician had wondered aloud how my body could tolerate this. But I had grown so used to living with the condition and managing its effects that I saw no urgency in rushing to surgery. So I thought I should allow the idea some incubation time and some planning. However, another health event occurred about the same time as my Cardiologist was telling me I should have my valves surgically repaired that hastened my agreement. It was to do with gum disease. In my late twenties my dentist had told me that my gums seemed to be receding 'a little', but it was nothing to worry about – yet. I saw his hygienist and was well primed in flossing and oral health. From then on I took especial care with my teeth and the issue never came up again for well over than twenty years. Then my gums started bleeding and after a few days it seemed to be bleeding even more, even though I used a good mouthwash designed for gum infection and took special care with brushing and flossing. I had not seen a dentist for over a year. I had decided to change dentists and had not yet got round to finding a new one. I phoned around my friends and found a highly recommended group practice and made an appointment to see the same dentist used by my friend. While waiting for the appointment, three of my lower front teeth began to wobble. More than anything else, this terrified me. My first appointment with the new dentist involved a very thorough examination and the photographs of the roots of the teeth I was shown left me speechless. The first question the dentist asked me after the examination was "do you have a heart condition?" When I explained my valve issues, he said, "You better have it fixed". Looking back now, I am surprised that he did not discuss the issue of inflammation generally, but I guess there is never time for everything.

My gums did stop bleeding some days after a thorough de-scaling by the hygienist and the wobbly teeth did eventually stabilize sometime after surgery to repair my valves. It is however hard to tell if successful heart surgery helped in any way to improve the health of my gums.

Chapter Five

My Joints Are a Moving Target

Well before the discovery of my prolapsed mitral valve, I began to feel pains in the joints on the right side of my body. First it was the right ankle, then the right knee and hip and eventually the shoulder. Frequently the pain and accompanying heat traveled from the shoulder, along the neck and radiated into the head, causing pain in the right ear. I had ignored it for a while. But the shock of the mitral valve prolapse diagnosis spurred me to action on that front. So the next time the pain flared up aggressively, I visited my physician and he made a referral to see a rheumatologist. My blood tests showed a moderately raised rheumatoid factor and in fact the rheumatologist that I may well have rheumatism. I was prescribed a non-steroidal anti-inflammatory (NSAID) and asked to return in three months for a review. Three months later the level remained static. In another six months, it was absolutely normal. The conclusion of the rheumatologist was that what I had was some arthritic pain but it was not rheumatoid. The pain did not go away however, and I was offered more NSAID, which I turned down. I moved on to explore alternative means of managing the pain. I returned to yoga, which I had given up under the pressures of raising a family and career demands. I had regular Swedish massage, and a course of acupuncture. I eventually saw an osteopath. All that helped to improve my sense of wellbeing. But the pain seemed to have become a faithful companion.

There was an occasion a couple of years before the pain began, when a total stranger told me he thought my right ankle was swollen. I had gone to see a professor of engineering on a university campus. When I entered his office he was seated at his desk at the far end of the room and he watched me as I walked towards him. As he rose to greet me and before I had introduced myself, he said ' I hope you don't mind me saying this but your right ankle is swollen'. I said I doubted it but looked at it anyway. He said he would investigate it if he were in my position. I thanked him for his concern and told him I would investigate it. We proceeded with our meeting and as I felt no pain, I did not think much about his comments after I left his office. What makes a professor of engineering, not of medicine, so quick to point out signs of a possible medical problem and why was I so nonchalant about it all? Was it perhaps our different stages of life that made our attitudes so different, me still young enough to be convinced of my invincibility despite my already manifesting medical problems and he, approaching retirement and more aware of the fragility of the human frame? More than twenty years on, I have often wondered if I should have pursued that conversation with him when he seemed so interested in doing so. Was it bashfulness on my part or dedication to a professional pursuit? What insight might he have shared that might have helped me tackle the problem sooner than I did? Although I was unaware of it at the time, my body was being swamped by inflammation and my joints were under attack. This fact became clear when some years later while visiting my grandmother during a humid summer month my knees literally seized up. I could not bend the right knee at all and I walked with difficulty, so much so that when she and I were taking a gentle stroll she lent me an old family walking stick to help maintain my balance. It came upon me without warning and it seemed to slowly recede without rhyme or reason. Within a couple of weeks I was again fully mobile.

Some considerable time after my struggle with the eye inflammation uveitis and after my HBV had been diagnosed, my joints suddenly flared up again with a vengeance. All my joints on the right side of my body including those in my toes and fingers and wrist were inflamed and the right ankle joint was particularly swollen. The pain and the burning sensation were severe; I could not sit, I could not sleep, I could not read because I could not concentrate. I had by then moved to a new city and my new physician referred me to a new rheumatologist. Blood test and ultrasound were done, some NSAID was prescribed and we settled into another pattern of regular reviews. Once again my rheumatoid factor was slightly raised, but only slightly. This new rheumatologist was very interested when I told him I have HBV and paused a little on the history of that. He told me, for the first time ever, that the HBV virus is associated with joint pain and was the likely cause of my joint pain, which he referred to as polyarthralgia. Polyarthrialgia simply means pain in many joints but gives no clue to its cause. Interestingly, when I told my hepatologist of this information, he seemed as surprised as I had been. He said he had never heard of HBV related joint pain.

I was referred to a physiotherapist and had twelve weeks of supervised exercises with her. It made no positive difference. The rheumatologist offered me a course of steroid injections to reduce the pain. But because of my horrific experience with the side effects of steroid eye drops, I declined it. He then prescribed me the drug hydroxychloroquine. Developed as an anti-malaria drug it has now been latched onto by drug companies as an effective treatment for arthritis. I accepted the prescription but did not take the drug for nearly four months after it was prescribed. I wanted to check with my hepatologist first, in case it was contra indicated by my liver disease. The hepatologist had no concernsand gave me the do ahead to take it., and so I eventually took the prescribed daily dose of the drug. I felt no positive effect on my aches and pains. However, within a few months of taking the drug hyroxychloroquine, I was experiencing pain inside both ears and I noticed that my hearing in the right ear was muffled. I was missing conversation especially where there was background noise. I stopped taking the drug and reported my symptoms to my general physician.

I was referred for an auditory test. The results confirmed that I had partial sensorineural hearing loss. My ability to hear faint sounds is very much reduced. Even where the speech is loud enough to hear it may still appear unclear or muffled. According to the audiologist my inner ear or cochlea has been damaged. I am told that it is damage that most of the time cannot be medically or surgically corrected. Not that I would choose to take another step to tamper with my hearing. The audiologist who saw me was very emphatic about stopping the hydroxychloroquine and never ever taking it again. He seemed very familiar with this atrocious side effect of the drug and said I should never have been prescribed it. It is what is known as an ototoxic drug. When I asked if there was anything that could be done to reverse the hearing loss, he said he didn't think so but that it was unlikely to get any worse after stopping the medication. I was offered a trial hearing aid which I have resisted using. I now know from my research that there are more than 200 drugs that are ototoxic. These are drugs that can damage the ear, cause hearing loss, ringing in the ear or balance problems. Although it is often claimed that hearing can be restored when treatment with the medication is discontinued, in many cases hearing loss is permanent. Nearly three years after I stopped taking the drug, I was given another hearing test and review. As the audiologist anticipated, there was no improvement in my hearing and there has not been since.

I also know that good practice requires that when a decision is made to treat a serious condition with an ototoxic medication, the doctor must consider with the patient the possible effect on her hearing and balance systems and how such side effects will affect her quality of life. Not only did my rheumatologist not do this, he also reacted with utter surprise when I reported this particular side effect and told him that I had taken myself off the drug as a result. He in fact said my loss of hearing was unlikely to have been caused by the drug. He seemed the only one among the doctors who care for one or other of my conditions who appeared surprised by my suffering this side effect. His inability to come down from his pedestal and concede to a patient that he made a mistake was perhaps not exceptional in his profession.

Hydroxychloroquine is used to treat lupus and rheumatoid arthritis as well as several other conditions. My rheumatologist had decided that what I have is neither rheumatoid arthritis nor lupus but an inflammatory condition arising from my HBV infection affecting multiple joints and described by the omnibus term polyarthralgia. Thus strictly speaking the drug had been prescribed to me 'off-label", that is to say it was approved for a different use from that for which my doctor prescribed it. Apart from the fact that it was of no benefit and in no way improved my condition, the rather serious side effects were never mentioned and explicitly weighed against the somewhat flimsy chance it might help me. Nor did I have a say in assuming such a serous risk. Should a highly placed professional be able to get away with such shoddy behavior? The likelihood of patients with multiple chronic illnesses being prescribed drugs off-label is much higher than one might imagine. Reflecting on this unnecessary addition to my list of chronic health conditions, I resolved that in the future I would avoid anything looking remotely like off-label prescribing of drugs. Chloroquine is a headline anti-malarial drug. But as its effectiveness as an anti-malarial drug has waned, other uses have been found by the drug companies by promoting other versions of the drug. Thus hydroxychloroquine now boasts a long list of established uses involving a daily dose. Yet it has treacherous side effects and the scenario is hardly different from off-label prescription.

I set out to gather information about the practice. What I found is concerning. When a doctor writes you a prescription, you may not know what the drug you are going to take was really approved by the FDA for. It may have been approved for use on a condition that is very different from the one you are being treated for. Apparently once a drug has been approved doctors do take the liberty of writing off-label prescriptions. In fact according to recent studies, as many as one in five prescriptions are written for off-label use – such as an epileptic drug prescribed for depression. This because what the FDA regulates is drug approval, not drug prescribing. Once a drug enters the market doctors may prescribe it as they think fit. Thus the practice is legal, if arguably unethical. But it is decidedly unsafe, even extremely dangerous. The pitching of drugs for unapproved uses has been a very common practice that has cost drug makers billions in fines over many years. Yet this unsafe practice still goes on all the time. Doctors learn about new, unapproved ways of using drugs from the reps of the pharmaceutical companies. Drug reps tell them a certain drug has been found to help or treat a certain condition. If the information catches on, it's a boon for drug companies, especially with drugs that have been overtaken by more recent discoveries in this age of disruptive biotechnology. The medical ethics advocate and assistant professor of medicine at the University of Chicago Medical Centre G. Caleb Alexander, MD, MS, has been quoted as saying: "doctors are free to prescribe a drug for any reason they think is medically appropriate. Off-label use is so common, that virtually every drug is used off-label in some circumstances." Some examples of off-label drug use promoted by drug reps are mind-boggling. They include dangerous anti-seizure medications given for headaches, depression and nerve pain, highly risky anti-psychotics prescribed for Alzheimer's disease or given to children for attention deficit hyperactivity disorder and autism. Beta-blockers approved for heart disease are prescribed for migraines and anxiety. Patients who are given these dangerous and powerful drugs do not know what they are intended to treat, especially given in times of crisis when they are vulnerable and very dependent on their doctors. Anyone who has chronic HBV is likely to also have other chronic medical conditions. Those of us who have chronic illnesses and especially multiple chronic illnesses need to be acutely aware of the huge risks we face when we undergo drug treatments for lengthy periods of time.

If, as in my case, you find yourself being prescribed multiple medications by different specialists, the risk you run of serious side effects and injury are multiplied. When any of the drugs are prescribed off-label, you may find yourself in great danger of developing other conditions that are purely induced by the interaction of drugs, or indeed by the prolonged use of single drugs. We thus owe it to ourselves to establish with our doctors that prescriptions handed to us are not off-label, or in the very least if a prescription is off-label, that the reasons for the decision to prescribe it is discussed with us and all possible side-effects weighed up and our informed consent given for its use. Most of us have the capacity to understand fully what risks we are assuming if our doctors do the professional thing and seek our informed consent. Some excellent doctors whose patient I have had the good fortune to be at one time or another have encouraged open discussion and are not afraid to be challenged. If your doctor feels threatened or irritated by your questions or doubts, you are entitled to walk away and find a less insecure or less arrogant doctor. You care about your own life and health more than anyone else. Take charge of it.

I have come full circle once again. As I write this, the autumn chill has set in. My joints are literally killing me and I have an appointment to see an orthopaedic surgeon about the deterioration in my right ankle. A recent MRI scan ordered by my general physician shows that there is extensive damage to the bone and ligament of the right ankle joint, and there is some bone protrusion. The bone protrusion is detectable to the naked eye and is something I had repeatedly pointed out to the rheumatologist. His opinion was that it was simply swollen and apparently ultrasound and CT Scans he ordered had not revealed this problem. In the mean time, a lot of time having passed, the original condition has deteriorated significantly. Thus while I still have all my joint pain and more, because I took hydroxychloroquine, I have added hearing loss to my list of chronic conditions.

Chapter Six

Clues and Childhood Illness

When we were growing up my brother, my sister and I heard the stories told so often that it now feels as if we saw it all happen. First, a seemingly innocuous small pox vaccination given me as a toddler, then a few days later an exceptionally high temperature and a general lethargy that seemed to get more pronounced over several days. It led to the first of many hospital admissions. Over time I gained the reputation among family and friends, neighborhood and school of being a sickly child. When I started school at the age of four I was the only child in the school who went home for lunch. This was to ensure my mother kept an eye on my nutrition. When my class started a project vegetable garden at the age of 7 I was not permitted to dig in the school garden or do anything considered strenuous physical activity at school, including running and some games activities. This remained the case as I moved up the school. I was remarkably skinny. Breathlessness was a problem on exertion and there were a handful of fainting incidents the aftermath of some of which I can recall vividly today as if it were an out of body experience.

Two haunting memories remain with me always. During my pre-pubescent years, fluid filled spots would periodically appear on my hands in between the fingers, especially at the base. I would pick at them and pull away the skin, discharging the fluid and exposing what seemed like perforated skin underneath. It was always the same. The skin underneath looked as if several pinpricks had created these little holes. The interesting thing is, the skin would heal over very quickly, within a few days, leaving no scabs or scars. In my mind this looms as such a feature of my childhood that when I recently asked my mother whether she remembered that and she said she didn't, I felt quite let down and disappointed. But then I might have buried myself in my own world and not showed it to the adults in my family. After all it did not cause any pain. The other memory was more of a drama. Aged nine, I had been in bed with a fever and flu symptoms for a few days and, feeling a little better, ventured on my own to the bathroom. I remember rushing out of bed thinking it was an emergency. I felt hot and heavy. However, as I sat on the loo, instead of a bowel movement there was a forceful rush of thick liquid into my mouth, literally forcing my mouth open and projecting itself onto the floor. There seemed to be bucket loads of it and my body followed it onto the cold floor of the bathroom. I remember feeling a sense of relief as I touched the floor and that is as far as my awareness went.

My mother takes over the story. She had got up from her desk which stood in a corner of the living room to stretch her legs. She thought she had seen me cross the corridor in her peripheral vision. She walked past the bathroom on her way out onto the terrace. The bathroom door was ajar and she noticed two skinny legs stretching out on the floor. No one had to tell her I was in a critical condition. She rushed into the bathroom and picked me up from a pool of blood and lumps of clotted blood I had expelled from my body. She rushed out of the house into the middle of the street followed by whoever else happened to be at home at the time so that no car could get by without stopping. They literally hijacked the first car that drove by. I was rushed to hospital apparently unconscious, cradled in her arms and both of us covered in blood. I spent several weeks in a large airy children's ward that I knew well from a number of previous admissions. I had apparently been kept in an emergency suite for nearly a week before that. I have little recollection of the emergency suite. I went home from hospital on my tenth birthday to a 'thanksgiving' feast. To this day, I do not know what caused such a dramatic collapse of my system. Nor did my mother, because apparently there was some conjecture, but no clear diagnosis.

There might have been a little clue to the puzzle about five years later. At the age of fourteen I had a fairly extensive medical examination because of a general feeling of fatigue, repeated fainting spells and rather extreme sport-induced breathlessness. I remember being told that I had a kidney infection and being prescribed some medication and recommended a salt-free diet. This was more than a decade before the HBV virus was discovered and named. When subsequently asked what illnesses I have had I would always mention a kidney infection. Yet I have been told there is absolutely no sign of anything having been wrong with my kidney. I remember the heavy German accented English spoken by the kindly elderly doctor who made that diagnosis. Did he really mean 'kidney', or had he intended to say 'liver'? I will never know for sure.

Chapter Seven

A Change of Heart

Five days after open-heart surgery to repair my badly prolapsed mitral valve and leaking tricuspid valve I returned home from hospital. I had hoped that I would have a minimal incision procedure but the surgeon explained that while it is straightforward to use a minimal incision for the repair of a single valve it was riskier with two valves. In his assessment, it was best not to make two separate incisions or enter the body twice on the same occasion. I was happy to accept his assessment. I had resisted any form of heart surgery for many years. I had complete faith in Dr C, my cardiologist and we agreed that he would monitor my condition and let me know when it was no longer sensible to delay repair surgery. In the intervening years I had taken exceptional care about my general health. I took my fitness to optimum levels for my age and ailments. I embraced nutritional medicine, yoga, pilates, long country walks and meditation. I learned to manage my energy and I coasted along just fine. I got on with professional work and although the burden of multiple chronic health issues nagged in the background, things were generally well enough and I looked forward to the future, albeit with some trepidation.

Some years down the line however, an ultrasound examination showed that my tricuspid valve had also started leaking, apparently a result of it taking over much of the work load of the mitral valve. There was some increase in the enlargement of the heart. It also seemed to pound louder and louder as time went by. I was increasingly breathless on minimal exertion and walking up long flights of stairs or going uphill could be a struggle. My quality of life was beginning to decline. There were other clinical indications of a need for intervention. Then the shocking news of a sudden death in my family sent me into a frightening fainting episode. I was unable to get up and walk and I was hyperventilating. I have no recollection of how I got to hospital. I only vaguely remember answering a doctor's questions while seated in a wheel chair that stood by his desk. The following two days passed in a haze. As I slowly regained my equilibrium I knew without being told, that it was time to sort out my valves. I was told that the shock could have killed me. I trusted and respected the opinion of my cardiologist who I had known for some fifteen years. And when he told me it was time to have the operation, I readily agreed.

In the event, when I had the pre-op angiogram, my arteries were found to be completely free of obstruction. The surgery itself was therefore very straightforward. The oxygen bypass procedure lasted 78 minutes. Recovery was equally without incident. The first dose of morphine I was given did its job so well that I was able to turn down a second dose when I was offered it in the intensive care ward. Immediately after the operation I was put on several drugs, including the dreaded blood thinner warfarin and one for atrial fibrillation. I raised many concerns with my medical team. I was assured I would be on the drugs for twelve weeks and no longer. I agreed, with reservation. Warfarin's list of possible side effects scared me greatly. Many of them are extremely serious. And as I had learned from my experience with maxidex, with drug side effects the reality can often be much worse or more common than claimed by pharmaceutical companies. The hospital pharmacist's review of the supplements I was taking and had been taking for a long time, in some cases for years, was interesting to say the least. In order to give warfarin the chance to work properly and in a way that could be properly monitored by regular weekly blood tests, I was asked to stop a number of nutritional supplements two weeks before surgery and throughout the period I would remain on warfarin. The logic made clinical sense. In the real world it seemed like topsy-turvy thinking: warfarin is a blood thinner and anti-coagulant. It is given to prevent blood clots forming in your arteries and causing a stroke. If you are taking anything else that also thins the blood, your blood may become so thin that you might suffer internal bleeding. We can monitor the effect of warfarin on the coagulation of your blood. But we cannot monitor the effect of your supplements. So stop taking your supplements which may be achieving the same result as warfarin". The dietary supplements I had to give up during the three-month period were vitamin E, coenzyme Q10, vitamin D3, omega 3 and vitamin K2, a complex of anti-inflammatory systemic enzymes containing ginger, turmeric, L-glutathione, some bioflavanoids and bio-glucans. Most were contained in a single multivitamin and mineral capsule. These supplements had helped put me in peak condition in readiness for surgery and I was dismayed to have to stop taking them a couple of weeks before the event. I believe it was because of taking the supplements that my arteries were found to be remarkably clean during my angiogram. And these are the very supplements that I needed to support my immune system and aid a swift recovery.

A Viral Maze

Thus when at my 12-week review appointment the surgeon suggested that I continue taking warfarin, my reaction was an emphatic no. When he suggested a daily dose of asprin because it would be "helpful" to me I had to disagree. Fortunately, my cardiologist seemed to agree I did not need any further heart medication. I was thus able to return to my dietary supplements, and the difference in my mood was almost immediately noticeable. However, it took much, much longer to regain my former energy levels and my lung capacity than I had been led to expect. But all is well that ends well. My six inch long badge of honor now graces my chest and I have promised myself to continue wearing the same tops I used to wear before the operation – mostly with scooped and V necklines, and not invest in new clothes. It has also given me the incentive to wear the many beads and necklaces I collected in my youth, a new addition to my wardrobe that during the summer months very successfully distract attention from my prominent scar.

Chapter Eight

It's Systemic Inflammation, Stupid

I have struggled throughout my life to make sense of my chronic lack of energy, childhood fainting spells, bouts of social withdrawal and hibernation, mental confusion and melancholy. These characteristics, however, seem to be at odds with what appears to be my innate personality during periods of good health. Even as a young child, I was conscious that there was an underlying reason for what I saw as my personal change of seasons. As an adult, I have tried at various junctures to interest my primary physicians as well as my specialists in helping me connect the dots. Not much interest has been shown. The oft-heard claim that the healthcare sector needs big improvements is now backed up by so many patient accounts that it is a trite assertion. A critical problem with healthcare is that it is often delivered as if the organs of our bodies are separate and independent one from the other, rather than the interconnected systemic whole that they are known to be. This makes the diagnosis and treatment of chronic illness often a hit and miss affair that seldom uncovers the real cause of the problem. At various stages of my early life, there were warning signs that pointed to a serious underlying illness. The clues were there for the knowing eye to see. Yet, even as one illness followed another, the possible links between them were never properly investigated. With the proverbial benefit of hindsight, the clues to an underlying link between the various episodes were not exactly hidden from sight.

What are the connections between mitral valve prolapse, uveitis, arthritis or polyarthralgia and HBV, not to mention attendant chronic fatigue and palpitations? It is a question that I kept turning over and over in my mind. I brought it up as often as I could, especially when I saw my specialist doctors. I was startled that nobody was seriously interested to connect the obvious dots. When I brought up some apparent connection one or other of them might say, oh how fascinating, and then move right on. I guess they have other patients to see and they are not research scientists. But are they not committed to doing their best for each of their patients? Would an integrated approach to healthcare not yield better professional as well as resource allocation outcomes? I concede that may not be as much a matter for individual physicians as it is a structural problem for the profession and its institutions. I had been particularly disappointed by the cursory contextual investigation that accompanied my diagnosis and treatment for uveitis. My otherwise excellent ophthalmologist was not interested in what she may well have considered to be a wild goose chase for the cause of the condition. In the main, she seemed content to keep repeating to me that there may be a number of possibilities but the cause is really not known. I now know that viral infection can lead to uveitis. Of course viral infection causes inflammation throughout the body. A virus as resilient and destructive as HBV causes a whole lot of systemic inflammation that affects other organs in the body beside the liver. When after my HBV diagnosis I came across this possibility in my research I put the question to my ophthalmologist at the time as well as a rheumatologist. Both of them said there was no connection between HBV and uveitis. Neither of them left open the possibility that there might be such a connection. When I changed ophthalmologists a couple of years later, I was lucky to have a very thoughtful lady professor. I asked her whether there might be a link between HBV and uveitis, she paused for a while then said 'the evidence is just beginning to come in from people who have received the HBV vaccine. It seems there could be a connection'. I very quickly relayed this information to my hepatologist at my next appointment to see him. He had not heard of the possibility of a connection. I brought it up again during my most recent appointment, three and a half years later. He still had heard nothing about it through his professional network. And I keep on wondering whether doctors in different specialties speak to each other systematically about their clinical research or experience. How long does it take for the multidisciplinary connections to spring into action? Is there a structured framework for information sharing and multidisciplinary discourse at the clinical level?

What I have learnt through all this is that nothing is more important in healthcare than a joined up approach to healing. As one grows older, when multiple chronic diseases tend to emerge, it is the height of folly, or perhaps hubris, for so many physicians and specialists to continue to treat patients as if the organs of the human body are wholly independent one from the other. While increasing numbers of doctors are adopting the multi-disciplinary approach it is far from a trend. For anyone suffering from multiple chronic illnesses it is important to find one of these imaginative and dedicated physicians and specialists. They are reassuring and may even have the humility to quietly recognize that other systems of medicine - the nutritional, naturopathic, complementary, osteopathic or functional, may have an important place in a multi-disciplinary approach to healing or managing our illnesses. Of course a conventional physician will not be in a position to point you in that direction. But they may at least refrain from rubbishing a patient's decision to explore them and will constructively highlight any possible risks to guard against. I have had the good fortune of finding such a doctor, after years of searching. When we enter the healthcare system with a serious condition we often do so with trepidation because we know we are in for a tortuous journey. Some things will probably go wrong. We will spend money on questionable diagnoses and treatments. We may learn little about the true nature and extent of our condition. We may come away with more illnesses than we started with. This is in spite of the fact that technology has made a quantum leap in the last decade and continues to march forward as better and better surgical procedures are developed and major advances are made in medicine. The working relationship between patient and doctor is critical and requires a good dose of professional humility and empathy. The journey of exploration that is necessary to uncover and treat the true cause of a serious illness requires true partnership and mutual respect. The capacity to really listen the patient is the hallmark of successful healthcare. For surely no one knows a patient's body better than the patient. I have been lucky enough to be cared for by doctors who practice their profession as a true calling. But I have also encountered doctors who seem to show little interest in really hearing and understanding what the patient has to say about how they experience their illness, whatever it may be. The real culprit in such cases is often the doctor-patient relationship.

After a tortuous lifetime's journey through the healthcare maze, I am now convinced that each one of my chronic conditions is directly linked to the others. The 'original sin', as it were, was hepatitis B. Systemic inflammation caused by the hepatitis B virus has been responsible for all my other chronic illnesses.

World Health Organization literature informs that the commonest cause of HBV in babies is transmission from the mother. Now in her mid-nineties, mine has been blessed with an incredibly healthy and active life. Her only chronic condition is the seasonal flare-up of a knee injury sustained in a school sport accident in her early teens, and in the last year, episodes of hypoglycemia. An experienced sleuth of the mysteries of my health, she is convinced that I contracted HBV as a toddler from a small pox vaccination, probably from a contaminated needle. It is more than likely that my mitral valve prolapse was caused by systemic inflammatory insult from the HBV, progressively weakening the valve muscle and making it unable to close effectively, initially with the mitral valve, and eventually also the tricuspid valve. The knowledge that viral infections do cause inflammation in the body has been established for some considerable period of time. There is also emerging clinical evidence, according to an ophthalmologist at a leading Eye Hospital with whom I have discussed the issue that the eye inflammation known as uveitis can possibly result from HBV infection, indeed possibly from the HBV vaccine. I have come to a firm conclusion that the cause of all my other chronic conditions has been HBV induced systemic inflammation. Throw into the mix the side effects of the steroid eye drops used to treat my eye inflammation, which led to aggressive premature cataracts in both eyes. Add to the mix also the hearing loss that has resulted from the treatment of my joint pain with hydroxychloroquine. The fainting episodes, altitude sickness, chronic fatigue and brain fog, all seem to be linked to my 'original sin' of contracting hepatitis B. Systemic inflammation is known to be linked to almost all of the degenerative conditions known to man, including cancer and Alzheimer's disease.

Rooting out my systemic inflammation, or in the very least managing it successfully, is obviously the way to go. Finding a cure for HBV would of course be better still, but one has to deal with the current reality. What is tremendously empowering is that the cause of my multiple chronic illnesses is no longer a mystery. HBV cannot yet be cured, but it can be permanently kept under control. With that knowledge comes a remarkable sense of calm. What a difference knowing makes.

Chapter Nine

Tomorrow's Promise

Huge advances have been made in the management of HBV in the past decade and antiviral drugs are having a big impact. Although there are still no treatments that can cure HBV infection, treatments can suppress infection and prevent the disease from progressing. We now have aggressive drugs such as Entecavir that can rapidly reduce the viral load and are resistant to viral mutation. The promise of biotechnology to provide cures for so many hitherto incurable diseases in the near future is also far reaching. Advances in these two areas are particularly promising. The future is extremely bright.

Personalized medicine will change the way hepatology, and indeed other areas of medicine, is practiced. The potential for the use of adult stem cells to cure HBV is being aggressively developed and is beginning to yield positive results. The developing field of epigenetics is likely to impact hugely on this area of medicine. RNA interference, a revolutionary therapeutic technology that allows a disease to be halted in its tracks by simply switching off an already expressed gene could have unimaginable effects on how the HBV virus affects our cells. Being diagnosed with HBV today throws up a very different set of circumstances from what it was twenty, even ten years ago. And with the expansion of the choices for treatment will come a greater role for the patient in the management and possible cure of the disease.

The promise of the emerging field of medical humanities and the concept of whole person care will increasingly question the propensity of the medical profession to separate the body into its parts and thus miss the forest for the trees. Happily there is evidence of a growing band of outspoken advocates within the medical profession itself that see the importance of a joined up approach to the treatment of the human body and mind, the sharing of points of connection and of difference. Together with the strident advances being made in biotechnology, a truly brave new world beckons for the HBV sufferer, for patients with multiple chronic conditions, and for patients everywhere.

Men Interviewed Tell: 101 Things Women do to Turn Men Off

Dr. Cassandra A. George Sturges
MA, MA

iUniverse, Inc.
New York Lincoln Shanghai

Men Interviewed Tell: 101 Things Women do to Turn Men Off

iUniverse books may be ordered through booksellers or by contacting:

iUniverse
2021 Pine Lake Road, Suite 100
Lincoln, NE 68512
www.iuniverse.com
1-800-Authors (1-800-288-4677)

Because of the dynamic nature of the Internet, any Web addresses or links contained in this book may have changed since publication and may no longer be valid.

The information, ideas, and suggestions in this book are not intended as a substitute for professional advice. Before following any suggestions contained in this book, you should consult your personal physician or mental health professional. Neither the author nor the publisher shall be liable or responsible for any loss or damage allegedly arising as a consequence of your use or application of any information or suggestions in this book.

ISBN: 978-0-595-46589-7 (pbk)
ISBN: 978-0-595-90885-1 (ebk)

Printed in the United States of America

To: Sidney & Michael with all my heart

Acknowledgement

Thanks Harry Lawrence for editing.
Thanks Sidney for the concept for the cover

Introduction

Before you commit to another diet, smooth on a new shade of lipstick, dye your hair another color or purchase a new outfit ... read this book to find out what really turns a man off.

Many women think that it is external, physical attributes that keep a man interested in them sexually. They think that if they are pretty enough, or have the perfect body, the man in their life will love them more. I was shocked to hear men confess to me the things that women do to turn them off. These conversations began just anywhere—at the local Coney Islands', in offices, bar rooms, gyms and just standing in line at the grocery store. Each story is a combination of many situations and is not specific to any one man that I interviewed. I promised anonymity to each male who unveiled his heart for this book.

Over 100 men interviewed share down-to-earth, heart-to-heart, soul-stirring revelations about the things that women do to deeply hurt, humiliate and turn men off sexually. This book is a must read for any woman who is serious about finding, keeping or creating a healthy, loving relationship with a man.

If you think that most men do not have feelings or that the main reason that a man is no longer sexually attracted to a woman is because of her physical appearance—This book is guaranteed to make you take a deeper look at yourself and discover some of the unspoken reasons that men leave relationships and are turned off by women.

1. Saying negative things about his mother.

"My mother is rude and controlling. I know this. But she is the woman who brought me into this world. When a woman criticizes my mother or calls her out of her name, I know that she is not the one for me. To me it's not an issue of love, but respect. Good or bad, she is the only mother I will ever have. When a woman disrespects my mother, it tells me who she is as a person and that we don't share the same family values."

2. Unable to get along with his family.

"Everybody knows that Uncle Joe is a fool. He doesn't mean any harm; he just drinks too much and talks too much stuff. He loves the attention of making everyone laugh. Uncle Joe told my girlfriend that if she didn't eat more food, a good wind would just blow her away. My girlfriend sulked all night. I tried to comfort her and Uncle Joe even apologized. It's been over a year and a half ago and she still claims that my family is ignorant and stupid. We are still together but I am slow to propose marriage to this girl because I am very close to my family. I feel that further down the line I would be forced to choose between my family and my wife. This is a situation that I don't want to be in. I figure that in time my girlfriend will learn to accept my family, or we will have to break-up to make room for my perfect girl to enter my life."

3. Flirting and acting seductively in the presence of other guys.

"I think that it is human nature to flirt, but giving the impression that you are available is embarrassing. My wife always says, 'Honey, you know I would never sleep with nobody else, I just like seeing guys get hot and bothered.' I worry that one day the right man is going to make her change her mind. I admit that I feel jealous and angry, but definitely not aroused by her. There's a lot of flack from male friends about how they can have my wife anytime they want to, some claim that they have already had her. I don't know what to believe. But I do know that it is difficult for me to want to be with her sexually, because of her open seductive behavior."

4. Depending on him to be financially responsible for her bills.

"A lot of women believe that it is a man's responsibility to pay their bills, finance their hair and nails and give them an allowance. I am single today because it is difficult to find a woman who acts like a responsible adult. I don't mind helping a woman in need, but it is not my responsibility to take care of a healthy, capable, grown adult. Hey ladies, have you ever heard of the word 'prostitute.' I believe that I could maintain a less expensive relationship with a whore. If you think that I must compensate you financially for a relationship then you need to determine if you want a John, a sugar daddy or somebody to love you."

5. Verbally attacking his ex-wife or ex-girlfriend.

"When my woman says negative things about my ex-wife, in essence, she is saying negative things about me. My ex-wife is a reflection of my taste in human beings. Just because things didn't work out between us, it doesn't mean that my ex-wife was all bad. Sometimes when I complain to my woman about my ex-wife, I just need her to listen and be supportive. But even when I ask for her opinion about a situation, all she has to do is to comment on the problem, not refer to my ex-wife using derogatory names. In the same way I wouldn't feel comfortable letting someone say bad things about *her* if we were to break up, because I will always love and respect her, whether we are together or not. When I try to tell her that I don't like it when she talks about my ex-wife, she accuses me of still having feelings for her. I do have feelings for her, but not sexual feelings of wanting to be with her in an intimate relationship. I wish she would give my ex-wife the type of respect that she would want someone to give her."

6. Being rude and disrespectful to wait staff, grocery clerks or other service help.

"My baby could give Halle Berry beauty tips. She is absolutely gorgeous until she interacts with someone who she thinks is beneath her. My secretary cringes whenever she calls, because she is so rude over the phone. We are not welcome in two restaurants because she insulted the waitresses and management there, by calling them stupid and ignorant. Guys envy me—until they have seen my girl in action. To be honest, she is so enticing to me that her rudeness to other people doesn't turn me off sexually, but I am sure as heck not planning to marry her. I couldn't deal with her snotty attitude for the rest of my life."

7. Getting pregnant in order to try to get him, or to keep him.

"Our marriage was at rock bottom so my wife decided to get herself pregnant, without telling me, by pretending to use her contraceptive when in fact she did not. When I realized what had happened I was of course very angry inside, but tried to say nothing. I just thought about having to keep going for the sake of the new baby and hoping that my wife would also join me in trying hard now to straighten things out between us so as to make the marriage work. She never really did that, and just thought that things should continue as before, but with an extra leash on me of another baby. It never worked out and things reached breaking point less than two years later. We separated and eventually were divorced. When women do this, they show themselves to be irresponsible and self-centered and having little consideration for the children that they bear"

8. Leaving him a list of things to do—or planning his daily activities.

"My wife would leave me these elaborate lists every Saturday morning of things to do around the house. This gets me infuriated with her. Who does she think she is to plan my day for me? I would never ever think of telling her what to do and how to spend her day. She may want to spend the afternoon having coffee with her girlfriends or getting her nails done. I try to be a good husband by supporting my wife, but she treats me like a child instead of an adult. She then wonders why I am not that interested in having sex with her that often. Well, I am not turned on by her parental attitude."

9. Dictating to him how he should spend his spare time.

"I never tell my wife when I am taking a day off work, because she'll look at it as an opportunity for me to be her slave for a day. Sometimes women don't understand that men can feel smothered in a relationship. Once we decide to commit to them they seem to think that we no longer have the right to spend time alone, or be with our friends or family without them. The thing that turns me off most about women, is that they don't value or understand the importance of spending timing alone to maintain a sense of self-purpose."

10. Telling him how he should spend his money.

"I can't buy myself a shirt without my wife complaining. I know that I am a good husband. I pay all of the bills. Hell, I don't even know how much my wife makes, or what she spends her money on. I still can't see the logic in women believing that the money she earns belongs to her alone and the money I earn belongs to her as well. If my wife would chip in on the bills I wouldn't have to work so many long hours."

11. Making him feel like he has to be somebody he is not, just to make her happy.

"I am from the south and sometimes I don't pronounce words as good as my wife think I should. I feel like I am always on guard to hide the simple-country-boy in me. She is always mad at me for not attending social events with her and her uppity friends. Whenever I decide to go, she complains all the way home about my grammar, not using the right fork and wearing the wrong tie. We been married 23 years and I still love who she is when nobody's looking. But I tell our boy, 'Son, if you got to pretend to be somebody else for her to love you, she doesn't love you 'cause she can't love who she doesn't know.'"

12. Pressuring him to marry her when he is not ready.

"I had two more years before completing my MBA after earning my bachelors. I wanted to get some experience in corporate America, and then start my own business in about 5 to 7 years. I told my girlfriend that she is the only woman I wanted to be with, but I needed to focus on stabilizing my career before considering marriage. This wasn't good enough for her, so she gave me an ultimatum to marry her or get out of her life. I was devastated, so I decided to marry her rather than lose her. We stayed marry about 6 months. She constantly complained about the hours that I spent studying in the library and making efforts trying to start a small business on the side. I said, 'Honey, this is why I wanted to postpone marriage until I got myself together financially.' She would insist that if I really loved her then she would come first in my life—not my stupid dreams. Biggest mistake of my life was marrying before I was emotionally and financially ready. Now when I meet a woman who is constantly pressuring me about where the relationship is headed, I immediately tell her 'nowhere' and then end the relationship. Marriage should only be the next step for two people who are whole and can stand alone, but chose to be together as equals in love."

13. Volunteering his services to her family and friends.

"I ain't bragging but I can fix damn near anything. My old girl was always volunteering my services to the neighbors and her friends to fix dishwashers, dryers, and so forth. She sent me to her best girlfriend's house to build a deck for her backyard. When it was time to pay, her girlfriend went into the room to get the money and came back buck-naked. Lord, I told that woman to put her clothes back on. The lady started crying and begging me not to tell my old-girl, her best friend. I agreed not to tell because the shock would have killed my baby to know her friend would stab her in the back like that. I don't think it's right for a woman to volunteer her man out to help other people without talking to him first about it."

14. Pouting. Not telling him what is really bothering her. Hoping he will guess and figure it out.

"Whenever my girlfriend is upset about something, she gives me the silent treatment and sulks around the house. I guess she wants me to beg her to tell me what's wrong. But this type of behavior gets the opposite response from me. I am not a mind reader. She is a grown woman who should know how to express her feelings. When women get in this mood, I usually leave the house. I can't stand to be around them. Women are always telling us to grow up, I think they should take their own advice sometimes about acting mature."

15. Constantly putting herself down. Complaining about her weight, hair etc ...

"Nothing is more unattractive than a woman who is disgusted with herself. Something about her spiritually is very unappealing. I don't notice stretch marks until they point them out to me. If men saw women through their own critical eyes they wouldn't be able to get an erection."

16. Disturbing him while he is watching a game or involved in a solitary activity.

"I wish women would get a life. Develop an interest in something other than pleasing other people. I don't care if it's watching soap operas. Find something to do that you enjoy, for whatever reason. If women could learn to cherish their own time alone, they wouldn't need to interrupt men whenever the man is busy and so isn't paying full attention to them."

17. Acting like his mother.

"If I don't want to eat vegetables ... so what? I am a grown man. Please don't smother me with criticism about my clothes, my friends and what to do with my life. I left home because I am a responsible adult. Just because I don't do things like you doesn't mean that it is wrong. I am looking for a mate, an equal partner, not a mother. My mother is irreplaceable anyway."

18. Constantly telling him how to dress and conduct himself in public.

"My wife hates my shoes. She hates the way I laugh. She hates the way I talk. I can't believe that she wonders why I don't tell her that I love her. I feel inadequate whenever I am with her. I prefer to stay home rather than be around with a woman who is embarrassed to be seen with me."

19. Threatening to end the relationship after the smallest argument or to manipulate the situation.

"Each time my girl breaks up with me, I leave a piece of my heart outside the door for protection. I stay with my girlfriend because I love her. But the truth is, I don't feel like the relationship is stable because every other week we're breaking up over some bull-crap. Constantly breaking up and getting back together has left my heart open to meet someone new."

20. Burning his clothes or destroying his personal property as a means of revenge.

"Slashing my car tires and bleaching my clothes doesn't make me regret staying out until 3 a.m. with my friends; it makes me regret the day that I ever laid eyes on her. I forgot about whatever the temporary argument was about: the permanent damage to my baseball collection—that I couldn't get over. My girlfriend would accuse me of loving material things more than her. That wasn't the issue; the issue was respect. If I am so horrible leave me, but don't destroy my belongings thinking that this is going to make me realize how beautiful, loving and sexy you are. It actually gets the exact opposite response."

21. Physically abusing him.

"I don't know what women think men are made of, but I have a news flash for you ladies … it hurts when you slap, kick, and hit us. I was raised not to hit women, but sometimes I have to fight my human instincts to protect myself when I am being physically threatened. I wish more women would tell their daughters to keep their hands to themselves. It's not endearing to be kicked in the testicles by an angry girlfriend."

22. Expecting him to read her mind.

"If a woman wants something in particular she should tell me. Women don't seem to understand that when a man truly cares about her, he wants to please her. We are not psychics. If you want something, don't expect us to guess or figure it out as an indicator that we love you."

23. Believing that he is responsible for making her happy.

"I hate it when my wife says 'I am bored honey, think of something for us to do.' Hell, why doesn't she come up with some ways to entertain herself? She should go back to school or do something else. It is not my place to make her happy."

24. Blaming him for her not living up to her full potential.

"My wife believes that it is my fault that we struggle financially. I am a social worker. I don't make a lot of money, but I love what I do. She wants me to be an attorney, so that I can bring home more money. She needs to get off her butt and go to law school. She quits her retail jobs every few weeks and goes long periods without working at all. But it's my fault we're poor. Yeah, right! Times have changed: a woman can have a career doing whatever she wants. Women don't have to live vicariously through men anymore."

25. Unrelenting criticism.

"Okay, I leave my socks on the floor. But when a woman constantly criticizes everything I do, I feel that I can't do anything right. So I stop trying altogether. Tip: If you complain about his driving, the way he pick his teeth and eats his cereal in the morning, all in one day, this is way too much criticism. When a man feels that he disgusts a woman in general, then this is the last woman he wants to make love to. Maybe have sex with, to relieve himself, but it's difficult to connect with a woman who thinks of nothing but what is wrong with you."

26. Not wanting him to spend time with his family.

"My wife and my sister never got along. Neither one of them realized how stressful this was for me. I would have to sneak my son over to my sister's house. I felt like I was cheating on my wife whenever I would go to visit my own sister. I saw both of their sides. They were both right and wrong. But in order for me to have peace after 12 years of marriage, I sided with my family during the time that my mother was dying. My wife refused to even go to the hospital to see my mother if she knew that my sister would be there. I wanted my wife to love me more than she hated my sister, but that could never happen."

27. Treating his friends rudely.

"My wife didn't ever speak to my friends when they visited my home. They don't visit me anymore because they don't feel welcome in my home. I have talked to her several times about referring to my friends as 'dogs and thugs.' They have never disrespected her and she has no reason to treat them this way. This turns me off from her. My friends will be there when she's gone."

28. Only putting an effort into her appearance when she is leaving the house.

My girlfriend can light up any room. I mean she is gorgeous. But when it's just the two of us at home alone, I am lucky if she takes a bath. Her hair stands up on her head, she wears this old baggy jogging suit with holes in it and she doesn't even brush her teeth. I am not saying that she has to put on a full face to be around me, but she could at least brush her hair together and bathe. Maybe even wear an old pair of fitting blue jeans around the house.

29. Make him feel like he needs to ask for permission to leave the house.

"Sometimes I feel like I just want to get away for an hour, just to be by myself. But whenever I leave the house without telling my 'mother', I mean my wife I get lectured. I think that for a relationship to work there should be some arrangement like: if I am gone longer than two hours and you don't know where I am, then if I am alive and not in danger I promise to call. Otherwise, respect a man for needing some space to collect his thoughts and be a grown-up. Geesh!"

30. Giving him a curfew.

"I don't see my friends very often, we get together maybe once a year. My wife tells me that my curfew is 2 a.m. in the morning, because nothing is open but legs, after this time. One year I came home at 4 a.m. We had been drinking beer, talking shit and remembering the good ole days. My wife threw all of my belongings over the front yard. I was humiliated. I love my wife, but sometimes I don't like her very much. And when I don't like her, I don't want her sexually."

31. Comparing him to previous boyfriends or husband.

"If he was so wonderful she should have stayed with him. Every person has good and bad qualities. When my ex-girlfriend told me that her previous boyfriend was a neat freak and the best kisser she ever had, she turned me off sexually. I am a sloppy person by nature, probably a sloppy kisser too. But I know that I am a good man and I treat her like a queen. I am not going to compete with her past, for her respect and love."

32. Throwing away his personal things that he likes, without his permission.

"I love to watch the football game in my raggedy underwear and socks with the holes. I feel raw and manly. I had these items since being a freshman in college. When I moved in with my girlfriend she took the liberty of throwing these things away without my permission. I felt like someone had gutted a piece of my soul, my history. She meant well, but somehow I feel like she disregards my relationship with my self, separate from her."

33. Not allowing him to have an opinion about how the home is decorated.

"My mother gave me a family heirloom, a century-old-grandfather clock. I asked my wife if we could hang it in the living room, as an honor to my family and so that my mother would feel proud when she visits. My wife refused to hang up the clock stating that it did not match the décor in the living room. This infuriated me. I pay all the bills, I let her buy whatever the hell she wants, but she can't find a way to add my family heirloom to the living room. Her selfishness turns me off. I still love her, even though, when I think about this, it rubs me the wrong way."

34. Telling his personal business to her friends.

"I overheard my girlfriend telling her female friend that I was having problems getting an erection. I was under a lot of stress on my job and we were heavily in debt. However, when I heard her sharing the most personal and intimate aspect of our relationship with her girlfriend over the phone, that dissolved something deep and special between us. I couldn't look her friend in the eyes knowing that she knew such intimate details. I was humiliated and felt betrayed by my girlfriend. She apologized, and we tried to make it work, but we eventually broke up. Sex was never the same for me after that."

35. Telling her mother or family about arguments and disagreements.

"Every time my wife and I get into an argument she calls her mother with the details. After we have kissed and made up, her mother is still angry with me. My wife gets angry with me because I don't want to go over to her parent's house to visit. Well, this is why. I don't want to feel uncomfortable because her family is still angry over the petty argument we had about who ate the last ice-cream bar a month ago. I always feel like it's me against my wife and her family."

36. Pretending that she doesn't care about what happens in the relationship.

"'You can do what you want to do. I don't give a hoot if you go or stay. My life will go on. As a matter of fact, I'll pack your stuff.' (Mocks girlfriend in a high-pitched voice) Cool, since she said that she didn't give a #$% about the relationship, I stayed at my friend's house for two nights. We drank, played cards and watched television. I came home and found my girlfriend crying on the couch with the same clothes on as when I had seen her last. Her face was swollen, hair standing up on her head. I was like—dang 'Girl, what happened to you?' She screamed, 'Fool, don't you know I love you? I called every emergency room and jail in the city. I haven't been to sleep. I was worried about you.' I was shocked to hear her say that she cared about me like that. I asked her to marry me six months after that happened. I felt good knowing that she would fight for our relationship."

37. Trying to change his behavior i.e. asking him to stop drinking, smoking, cheating etc …

"If I were a woman, I would leave a man who cheated on me or displayed other behaviors that I don't like. The stuff that women are willing to put up with, hoping that we will change, does not make us love or respect them more. It actually causes us to lose respect for them. When we change our behavior and clean up our act, the last woman we want to be with is the one who tolerated our bad behavior. Most men will look for a woman who would not have put up with that behavior, and who reminds us of our better selves."

38. Making negative references to his masculinity.

"If you were a real man, you would … blah blah blah. I couldn't open a jar once and my girlfriend acted like I didn't have a penis. She thought it was funny. I have a good sense of humor, but if I told my girlfriend that if she were a real woman she would have bigger breasts, she would never forgive me. I am a real person who happens to be of the male gender. I never feel more like a man than when I am making love to a woman. But if she can't see this, outside of having sex, then I'd rather have sex within a meaningful relationship where I feel less vulnerable as a whole person."

39. Reminding him that she doesn't need him, and what she could do for herself.

"I had this one girlfriend who would constantly tell me, 'I don't need you. I work every day. I can pay my own damn bills.' (Mocks female voice.) Each time that we had the slightest disagreement, she would go there. I feel like that what she was really trying to tell me was 'You are skating on thin ice—I could leave you in a heartbeat. I don't need you physically or emotionally.' Since she could do just fine without me, I left her. No, I didn't want her to need me; but I wanted her to want to be with me because she loved me."

40. Clinging to him while in public.

"My wife will not leave my side to go to the ladies room. She holds on to my arms as if she is afraid that I am going to dump her for someone else. I feel smothered. I can't even have a one-on-one conversation with a male colleague; I can forget about the female species. Her insecurity is such a turn off to me."

41. Using sex to manipulate the relationship.
(This is an overwhelming male response.)

"Ladies please don't use sex to punish us for not putting the toilet seat down, paying your bills or buying you a gift. I know my wife is pissed off when she turns down my sexual advances. Her sex drive is naturally higher than mine, so when she turns me down, I automatically know that I did something to make her angry. I enjoy making love with my wife because it feels good. Sex should not be used as an incentive for good behavior. If I have to earn or pay for sex, I would rather have it with a professional prostitute where I don't have to worry about pleasing her sexually."

42. Poor hygiene.

"My wife is angry with me because I seldom give her oral sex. We literally fight about this all the time. I don't know how to tell her this, but she doesn't smell good down there. She smells like fish. Even when she takes a bath her vagina has an odor that nauseates me. The first time I went down on her, I swear … I almost fainted. I literally went to the bathroom and threw up. Before marrying my wife, there was this one girl I dated who smelled like a rose down there. She had excellent hygiene. She took baths every night and took showers in the morning. I could lick her from her head to her toes. Maybe girls need to put more effort into their hygiene because of the way their bodies are made. I don't know, I am not a doctor."

43. Nagging.

"My advice to women is, if you told me the first time, and you know that I heard you, please don't repeat the request. Let the garbage run over until I trip over it. Let me see the consequences of my behavior. Telling me over and over again only makes me feel rebellious. Action speaks louder than words."

44. Letting her appearance go to hell once she feels comfortable in the relationship.

"I think that women don't want to accept that there is a difference between being in love with a woman and being sexually attracted to a woman. I love my wife and I would never leave her for another woman, no matter how much I am physically attractive to her. When I met my wife she was 150lbs smaller than she is now. Although, I am still very much in love with her, I am no longer sexually attracted to her. My wife has a beautiful personality and a beautiful soul, when I make love to her this is what I think about. But we don't have sex very often, because the physical, carnal part of my manhood is not always physically aroused by my wife's body. I would tell women that though you don't need to look like a supermodel or be perfect or skinny, for a man who loves you to be attracted to you, however, taking care of your physical body is sexually stimulating to a man and not doing so can be a great turn off. On the other hand, no matter how beautiful you are physically, when a man is turned off by who you are on the inside, it is almost impossible to get an erection."

45. Making him the center of her universe.

"I couldn't believe it, that my first wife would get upset with me for not going to the hair salon and grocery shopping with her. I felt that I couldn't breathe while I was married to her. I used to tell her, 'Get a life. Find something interesting to talk about other than what is on television.' We argued constantly because she had no one else to spend time with. She had no hobbies, no friends, no job, ultimately no personality."

46. Calling excessively.

"I had a girlfriend who called me everyday all day long. She wouldn't give me a chance to return her phone calls. I thought, man … if this girl is this desperate and lonely for someone to talk to, there is no telling what is wrong with her. I mean, didn't she have some female friends or somebody else to talk to? My family started teasing me. They referred to her as my psycho girlfriend each time she called. Maybe I am a little old-fashioned but I believe that to most men, there is something alluring about a woman who waits for the guy to do most of the calling. If a woman finds herself calling a man all the time, I would warn her to give him a chance to think about her and take action to find out how she is doing. The less a man has to do get a woman, usually, the less he is interested in her."

47. Not demanding that he respects her.

"I had a girlfriend who I only called when I wanted to have sex or needed money. I knew this chick was crazy about me. All the guys thought that she was the finest girl in high school. She was built like a brick shit house, long, thick hair and flawless, caramel skin. Good lord, she was sweeter than honey! But the girl didn't have an ounce of self-respect. The first time we had sex, I told her that I was seeing two other girls and that I didn't have time for a commitment. She insisted that I let her perform oral sex on me at that very moment. We had sex all night. She made me breakfast in the morning and gave me money for lunch. She assumed that giving me her love and money would force me into respecting her and wanting to commit to only her. It's almost like, say you go to a college and you never study and they just give you a college degree. Not only would you not have respect for the school or degree, you wouldn't tell anybody that you attended school there. This is what it is like when woman allows a man to use her and disrespect her. As a man, I can only value a woman as much as she values herself."

48. Taking him for granted.

"I think that the most important pair of words that a woman can say to a man is 'Thank you.' What turns me off is a woman who thinks that it is my job and responsibility to open the door for her and take out her garbage. These are not requirements. These are gestures of kindness. Just like saying thank you is a gesture of kindness. I wish more women were gracious."

49. Not treating his children from a previous relationship with respect.

"I dated this woman whom I wanted to marry, but I couldn't because it was obviously that she hated my children. I never told her why I kicked her out of my house and my life after three years of dating. I couldn't bring myself to tell her, because I knew that she couldn't force herself to love my children. She would only pretend to like them in my presence, if I told her why I couldn't be with her. This type of relationship would ultimately hurt my children's self-esteem. The way a woman responds to my children is the biggest indicator to me that will determine if I can seriously date her or not. She doesn't have to love them, but at least treat them with courtesy and respect."

50. Controlling when or if he can see his children.

"My ex-wife controlled me with our children. Whenever I wouldn't do whatever she wanted me to do, she threatened to never let me see my children again. I see my children every other weekend, but that's not nearly as much time as I want to spend time with them. She constantly tells the children that I am worthless. I can't stomach the way she holds my children hostage to control me. I dated this one girl who treated her children's father, the way my ex-wife treated me by using their children as pawns to control the resources in the relationship. I told her that she didn't know how much this hurts a man when a woman uses the children against their father. She told me to mind my own business. I *had* to leave her. Being with her was like taking a round trip to hell. Women expect men to pay child support, but they don't think that we have a right to spend quality time with our children without their say so. Women should take a look at themselves too, when wondering why there are so many single mothers in the world."

51. Saying negative things about him to his children.

"My mother use to always tell me what a low-down, dirty, scoundrel that my dad was. Deep inside, when my mother said these negative things, I felt that she was talking about me too, because I looked just like my dad and we had a lot of like ways—good and bad. My wife tells my son that he has a temper, just like his daddy. This really bothers me. I have told her several times that I don't like it when she says negative things about me to our son. She refuses to stop. She's a good woman, but this is the one thing that she does that really makes me angry with her. Sometimes I don't speak to her for days because I don't want to say the wrong thing. You know, men have feelings too."

52. Calling over to friends, relatives and neighbor's houses looking for him.

"My pager buzzes all night when I am out with my friends. If I turn it off, my wife accuses me of sleeping with another woman, and when I come home my clothes are strewn over the front yard. She calls my relatives and friends looking for me. She even asks them if I am cheating on her. It is so embarrassing. She thinks that the reason that I don't want to have sex with her is because I am cheating on her. It never crosses her mind that I am ashamed of her behavior, so too angry to even think about having sex with her."

53. Constantly bringing up past arguments.

"I tell my wife, how the hell can we work on the future when we can't get over the past? Whatever happened a year ago, or two days ago, can never be undone. We have a horrible relationship because my wife lives in the past. I am planning my future with another woman who lives in the present. My wife probably won't even notice that I am gone."

54. Excessive jealousy.

"If I turn my head, my wife accuses me of looking at another woman. She swears that I am sleeping with the girl on my job. I don't know why she is so damn insecure. She has a body that most women would die for. She must think that she is some hideous, unlovable monster, to think that I would want to lose her for anything in a skirt. What's on the inside of her is so rotten that it spoils the outside of her. I think the sexiest quality that anyone can display is confidence in her own worth."

55. Telling him that he needs to talk about the relationship.

"Whenever my girlfriend tells me that she needs to talk about the 'relationship,' I run for the hills. I feel like she is pressuring me to give her more than what already exists. Usually, we are getting along great until she wants to analyze why we're getting along. Talking about the relationship doesn't improve it from my perspective. Being happy with her is what makes me want to ask her to marry me. I would tell women that if the relationship is going great, this is not the time to scare the man away. Be still, keep being yourself and let him come to you … sort of like catching a butterfly."

56. Being constantly late for appointments.

"I know that you ladies go through a lot to get dressed, but so do we men. I go through great efforts to pick you up on time to show you how much I respect you. If I told you that I would pick you up at 7 pm, but arrived at 10 pm, you would be beyond pissed. When I go to pick my woman up, and she is not ready, I am completely turned off for the rest of the night. I don't like rushing through traffic and stepping over people at the theater late, trying to get to my seat. Women shouldn't take for granted what men go through to get there on time. We try to be on time because we care, not because we are super human beings and have less to do to get ready."

57. Whining

"'It's hot outside.' 'I have a headache.' 'I don't feel good.' My wife will keep saying the same thing over and over again, knowing damn well that it is nothing that either one of us could do about it. She whines constantly, like a little kid begging to buy candy off the ice-cream truck. She doesn't know how many times I have wanted to leave her, because I simply can't take her constant whining."

58. Telling him how to do a task.

"My wife asks me to wash dishes, then gets angry with me for not washing them the way she wants me to. So now, I don't bother to wash dishes. I am damned if I do and damned if I don't. As long as the freaking dishes are clean, what difference does it make that I don't stack the dishes the way she would. It may seem like it's an argument over dishes, but it is really about feeling appreciated for who you are. Women don't see how their being petty and picky over little household chores ruins the sexual passion in their relationships. They blame us for not helping out, but when we do, it is not good enough."

59. Not appreciating the little things that he does for her.

"I bought my girl three long stem roses and a little teddy bear for Sweetest Day. She thanked me, but could not stop talking about the diamond tennis bracelet her ex-boyfriend bought three years ago. Man, I had just gotten my car out of the shop and my student loans were kicking my butt. I didn't have money for gas to get back and forth to work because I spend it on her. No matter how much it cost, a woman should always show sincere gratitude when a man gives her a gift. Needless to say, we broke up two weeks later. I didn't want a woman like her hanging around when I became financially stable."

60. Talking to him as if he were a child.

"'You better be home by 12 A.M.' 'You'd better not let me catch you drinking beer with your friends.' 'You'd better have the yard racked by the time I get home from work.' Who died and made my wife boss? Geesh. I was better off living at home with my mother. Being married is like living in boot camp to me. Hey, you know people think married people stop having sex because of physical reasons. I don't think that's true. For me, my wife and I rarely have sex, because we don't treat each other like two people madly in love, but two people who are trying to run a household. The relationship has become too practical."

61. Asking a question when there is only one reasonable answer.

"'Do you love me?' 'Do you think I am fat?' 'Do you think I am ugly?' 'Do you think she is more beautiful than me?' I feel trapped when my girlfriend asks me these asinine questions. She knows that there is only one correct answer that any nitwit would get right. When I ask her why she asks me such ridiculous questions, she says that it's not my answer, but the way that I answer her question that's important to her. Hell, if you need to ask a guy these types of questions to determine if he really loves you,. I would guess that the relationship is in trouble. I don't like it when I feel like I am being interrogated and no matter what I say I am already guilty. Give a guy a break. Judge me by how I treat you."

62. Not being responsible for her own sexual enjoyment.

"When a woman lies in bed waiting for me to give her the orgasm of her life, I know that my work is cut out for me. Show me what you like and how you like it. Trying to guess and figure out what a woman wants can be a huge turn off."

63. Comparing him to her friend's or sister's boyfriend or husband.

"I could tell that my wife had a crush on her best friend's husband. He was making a load of money, drove a fancy car, and looked like he had just stepped out of a QG Magazine. She badgered me to go back to school to get a business degree because this guy had a business degree. She would buy me clothes similar to this guy's. This pissed me off with her. I had to let her know that I enjoy my work as a teacher. I don't make a lot of money but I love my job. I told her that the next time that she compares me with this macho guy, I am out the door. Period. The relationship is okay, but I know it's not going to last, because one, I am not good enough for her; and two, I don't want to be with someone who doesn't appreciate me the way I am. I think we both are secretly making do with each other until the right person comes along."

64. Saying 'yes,' when she means 'no,' just to please him.

"Ah man, there is nothing I hate more than to see a lady cry. It rips my heart apart. I was making love to this girl, you know, and I am enjoying it. I think she is enjoying it too, but when I look down at her, her face is all wet. At first I though it was just sweat. Then I notice that it was coming from her eyes. I was like 'baby, what's wrong, am I hurting you?' She just blurted out that she wasn't ready yet to have sex with me. She said that she thought that if she had said no, that I would never want to go out with her again. I don't want to take advantage of anyone. My momma raised me to respect women and most of all to respect myself. I don't want a woman who doesn't have a strong mind, you know, one that doesn't believe in herself. I mean this type of women, to me, is the type of person who wants to make other people responsible for her happiness."

65. Calling his mother, as if he is a little boy, to have her reprimand him for something he has done or said to her.

"I love my mother but it is not her place to referee arguments between my wife and me. When I told my mother to stay out of our business, she told me to tell my wife to stop calling her every time we have a disagreement. I told my wife to please stop telling my mother our problems, but she still does. I think she enjoys listening to my mother tell me, 'You better treat that girl right. You are lucky to have somebody who wants to take care of you and my grandkids.' I guess this is not a major turn off, it's just so irritating."

66. Not trusting him.

"When a woman let a man know that she doesn't trust him, that man knows that he has a license to do whatever he wants to do. My ex-girlfriend use to tell me that she couldn't trust me because 'boys will be boys.' I started to see myself through her eyes as some slithering liar, ready to pounce on the first woman who said hello. I was like … wait a minute. I have always been an upfront guy. I learned a valuable lesson from that relationship. You will jump through hoop after hoop trying to convince that person that you are trustworthy. But if a person doesn't trust you, it's because they don't trust themselves. I found out that my ex-girlfriend was having an affair with a guy in her class. When I confronted her about cheating, she said, 'I was just beating you to the punch. If you weren't cheating now, you were going to cheat eventually so what's the big deal.' Trust is more about how that person feels about themselves, not the man."

67. Not supporting his goals, dreams and purpose in life.

"I tried to start my own business, but my wife wanted me to get a government job with a pension. I would try to explain to her that I have always wanted to own a restaurant, but she said that I was ruining my family's future by trying to fulfill my dreams. I stopped sharing with my wife what is really on my heart and mind, because I know that she is not going to support it. I feel like when I share my ideas with her, she poisons them by not believing in me. There is a major rift between my wife and me because I have to pretend to be somebody else when I am with her. Our marriage is sad to me. I feel that I must choose—my wife or my dream. For now I have chosen my marriage *and* my dream; but I don't know how much longer that is going to last. I love my wife, but I am happiest when I am pursuing my dream."

68. Loving him for his potential as opposed to who he is right now.

"I dated this girl who wanted to be with me because I was in law school. I hated law; I just wanted to be like my father. I decided that I wanted to buy some property and open a record store. My girl started tripping out. Her entire attitude towards me changed. 'What am I suppose to tell my family and friends when they ask me about you. Should I tell them that you're some slum lord with a corner store?' she screamed at me one night. I was floored when she said this, because I thought she loved me for me, whether I was a taxi driver or a doctor. How would a woman feel if she met a guy who told her that he loved her for the potential perfect body that she would have if she worked out every day. Huh? When I meet a woman and I get the feeling that she is only interested in who I might be and what I might have in 10 years, I say the hell with her; I want somebody who loves me right now the way I am."

69. Trying to control him or change his behavior in general.

"I love to play basketball with my friends on Saturday mornings. I eat two bags of candy a week and I love to watch television for about an hour before bed. These are all things that my ex-wife hated about me. I hated the way she left her panty hose around the house and snorted while scratching her ear. None of these habits made me want to change her. There were too many good things about her for me to complain about behavior that I found annoying. I don't think it's fair to try to change a person's behavior if it doesn't hurt themselves or another person."

70. Demanding that he 'talk' before she is willing to open up emotionally.

"I had been dating this girl for a couple of months and she needed to 'talk.' I knew where this 'I need to talk' was headed. Sometimes I feel like women don't give men enough time to decide where the relationship is going. When I go out with a woman, I am not anywhere near thinking about marrying her by the second third or fourth month. I am still getting to know her before I can determine if, or what type, of commitment I want. Early in a relationship, I am not ready or able to expose myself emotionally, because early in the relationship I am not emotionally attached to the woman. When a woman wants to know, before I know, this is a definite turn off for me."

71. Badgering him for sex by calling him homosexual or accusing him of cheating.

"I know that women think that men are ready for sex at any moment, but this is not true. I have been working doubles, seven days a week, so I am totally uninterested in anything other than sleep. My wife accuses me of being a homosexual or having an affair because I am too tired to have sex. Why does she have to go there? Why has a man got to be a fag or an adulterer just because he doesn't want to have sex? Something about this seems so mean spirited to me. When I am in the mood for sex it won't be with her. I don't think women understand that men actually have feelings."

72. Loving her wallets more than him.

"Women always accuse men of wanting them only for sex. Well I think women are just as guilty for wanting men for what they can buy for them. It's a nice gesture for a woman to offer to pay for a meal every now and then. I had a girlfriend who wouldn't even put 50 cents in the parking meter."

73. Snooping through his personal belongings.

"I bought an engagement ring for my wife before we married and hid it in a secret box where I keep my journal, nude pictures of some of my ex's, and other personal things, tucked away in my closet. My wife, who at the time was my girlfriend, had a key to my apartment. I trusted her very much. I never imagined that she would go through my personal things while I wasn't home. While looking in my secret box, I noticed that it had been tampered with. I knew instantly that my girlfriend had gone through my things and I wanted to kill her. I felt embarrassed for her to know such personal things about me. I was angry because she violated my privacy. I decided that I loved her too much at that time to break up with her, but I sure as hell was not going to marry her. About four months later my girlfriend accused me of proposing marriage to someone else. She admitted that she found the engagement ring and that she was lucky to discover what a scum I had been. I told her that I knew that she had gone through my things and decided that I didn't want to marry her. We argued about the issue of privacy, but we got over it and married 18 months later. I forgave her, and we are doing great now, but this almost cost us our relationship."

74. Accusing him of being sexually attracted to her friends.

"'Do you think so and so is cute, do you think such and such got a nice body?' Why do women constantly ask us what we think about other women, then get jealous when we admit they are attractive? Don't ask if you don't want to know the answer. If she looks nice to you, then she probably looks nice to me. Just because another woman looks attractive it doesn't mean that we want to go to bed with her. I have spent nights arguing with my wife because she has accused me of looking in her friend's cleavage. We should have been making love. Women should stop bringing other women into their bedrooms and lives. To tell you the truth, there have been many times that I wouldn't have noticed her girl-friends in the least bit if she had not brought what they were wearing to my attention.

75. Cheating on him.

"I could put my head on a chopping block because I know this man had sex with my wife two years ago. I have no tangible proof, but it's something I know, like I know my first name. My wife made dinner and ironed my work clothes before she left home that day. There was something peculiar about her behavior, but I can't put my finger on exactly what it was. We were getting along just fine, at least from my perspective. The sex couldn't get any better. She told me that she was going to a function for her boss. While she was gone a neighbor called to tell me that he had seen my wife go to a motel with one of her male co-workers. I confronted my wife when she came home and she denied it. She cried. She called her friends to come over and vouch for her that she was at the party. They came over and stated that she was with them. I listened. But, I knew in my heart that they were lying. Since that day, I have not been able to obtain an erection for my wife because I know someone else has been there. We have had our ups and downs since then. We are still together and she is just as beautiful as she was the day I met her. But, I can't get over her cheating on me. I believe that if a man truly loves a woman and is tuned into her emotionally, he can sense when she has been unfaithful."

76. Not keeping the house clean.

"Her house smelled like dog poop. She had dirty dishes in the sink all the time and her kitchen floor was so sticky and dirty that it would literally pull my shoes off my feet. But, the girl was fine as hell. She kept her body clean and if you saw her on the streets you would have thought that she was a neat freak. We dated for three months before I got a chance to come into her house. I was shocked. I couldn't believe that she actually lived there. I was already taken by her by the time I saw her house. I didn't want to break up with her, but I knew that the relationship couldn't go any further because I didn't want children by a woman like this. We recently broke up because she wanted more from me than I could give. I refused to eat at her house or spend the night. She was a sweet girl, but I knew that I couldn't spend the rest of my life with somebody that nasty."

77. Not keeping the children clean.

"I don't mind dating a woman with children from a previous relationship. My mother was a single parent and we couldn't have made it without my stepfather. I am happy that another man was willing to step up to the plate and help my family survive. I dated this girl for three years, who had five children. I loved those kids they were as sweet as pie. The oldest child was 10 and the youngest was 18 months when we first met. I moved in with her and paid all the bills. No problem. I wanted her to get off welfare and go back to school to get her nursing certificate. Overall the relationship was good, but the children looked like little bums. She didn't comb the girl's hair. They went to school with their hair matted to their little heads. They wore dirty socks with holes in them. She didn't bother to iron their clothes and she seldom did laundry. I was embarrassed to pick the kids up from school. I started ironing the kid's clothes and my mother would come over to do laundry for us periodically. When my mother would come over to help with the children, this would piss my girlfriend off. She thought that my family was criticizing her and didn't think that she was good enough for me. She resisted my family helping her. She reminded us that those were her children—only. We broke up, about 4 years ago. I still see the children and spend time with them. I buy them gifts for their birthdays and Christmas. What I like about the young lady that I am dating now is that she treats her nieces and nephews great. We took them to the amusement park for a weekend and she kept the children immaculate. I know I am going to marry her."

78. Being financially irresponsible with her life. "Hey, don't worry about the money I earn, why don't you get a job."

"I can't believe the nerve of some women. This woman had the audacity to criticize how much money I spend on electronic equipment and fixing up my car. So? It's my money; that I work for. This chick didn't even have a checking account. Her paycheck was being garnished by every department store dumb enough to give her credit; and her parents were paying half of her rent to keep her from being evicted. She said that she didn't make enough to pay her bills, but every time I saw her she had a new outfit on. 'Okay; now you are telling me how to spend my money for our future.' What future? My bills are tight. I work long hard hours to buy what the hell I want to buy with my money. I have a house that I am paying the mortgage on. When I meet the right woman that I want to build a future with, then I'd be interested in spending my extra money on an engagement ring not some woman who is going to ruin me financially, just like she has ruined her own finances."

79. Not respecting her parents.

"I am from the old school. You know, the bible says, 'Honor they father and thy mother.' This is a basic part of my value system. I know my parent's aren't perfect, but they deserve my respect because they gave me life and brought me into this world. My ex-wife hated her parents. Both of her parents abused drugs and their rights were terminated when she was a little girl. Her aunt adopted her so she never lost contact with her parents. We went to my ex-wife's family reunion and her parents were there. They appeared to be still using drugs. They were both filthy and they were going around asking people for money. I felt sorry for her parents. When my ex-wife saw them, she told them that they were despicable, crack-heads who didn't deserve to be alive. She told them that their very presence was living proof that there is no God. She told them that worthy, good, decent people die everyday, while creatures like them continue to roam the earth. She said this in front of the entire family. Two days later her maternal grandmother had a heart attack. The entire family was in total disbelief that she would say this to her parents. We divorced fours years later. I would be lying to you, if I told you that this incident did not play a role in my wanting to leave her. There was something cold and vengeful in her soul and I knew that if I rubbed her the wrong way, she would spit the same venom at me."

80. Always arguing with somebody over some petty issue.

"Two words: Drama Queen. Uh huh. She can't go to the grocery store without arguing over something. She can't get along with the people on her job. Everybody is jealous of her for something or another. Of course she is always right. Yep, I had enough of that woman. Nothing turns me off more than a woman who seems to not know how to get along with other people and always has a gripe to grind with somebody."

81. Dirty finger and toenails.

"I know this may seem small-minded, but when I see a woman with dirty finger and toe nails I think she is nasty. Anybody can throw some deodorant up under their arms for appearance, slip on some lipstick and make it look good. But a woman has to be particular about herself, to pay attention to the details of her hygiene. I don't want a woman with dirty fingernails cooking for me. I get to think that other hidden parts of her body are unclean as well. This is a definite turn off for me."

82. Dirty dishrags.

"Dirty dishes equal roaches. Everybody has to eat. You know food nourishes the body. I think it's kind of spiritual for me. Dirty dishes in a house to me, are like wearing dirty underwear. I think it's the most basic chore that should be done in a house. I'll wash the dishes my damn self, but if this is a habit for her, I am out the door. This is one of my quirks."

83. Poor dental hygiene—yellow teeth.

"People say the eyes are the window to the soul, but to me it's a person's smile. Have you ever thought that a person was unattractive until you saw them smile? I don't care how shapely a woman is or how pretty her facial features are, if she smiles and her teeth are yellow, I have no further desire to get to know her. The thought of kissing that person is absolutely repulsive. I am also turned off by women who have teeth missing and rotten teeth in their mouth. To me it looks like a person who doesn't love or respect themselves. I think that people should invest in their own health and well-being, and dental hygiene is a sign that tells me how much a woman cares about her self."

84. Negative attitude about life in general.

"Nothing is ever right to my wife. She hates her job. She is always complaining about what's wrong. Everybody is ugly in her opinion. She is the most negative person I know. We have been married 12 years and the last two of those years we have not had sex. She thinks it's because she had put on a few pounds. Hell, that ain't it. I think she looks good. It's her cotton-picking negative attitude that pushes me away from her. I can't remember the last time that she had something nice to say about anybody."

85. Constantly asking him, "Do you love me?"

"You know why I don't call my wife during the day while I am at work? Because I know that she is going to want to get into this emotionally heavy conversation. She is going to ask me 'Do you love me?' Well of course I love her. Why do you think I work so hard to give her the things that she wants and needs? Every year I take her somewhere special, like a little honeymoon. We go out to dinner at least once a week. I come home straight from work, help around the house. I try to show my affection my kissing her on the forehead and hugging her. Maybe I am missing something here. I feel like when she keeps asking me every blasted day, 'Do you love me?' this is her way of saying that what I am doing is not good enough for her. Hell don't keep asking me if I love you, sit down and be fair to me and look at how I treat you. Don't I act like a man who loves you?"

86. No tact … picking arguments in front of his friends and family.

"My girl loves to show her butt when other people are around. I think she gets a kick out of humiliating me. This girl wouldn't know class if it jumped up and smacked her in the face. I keep telling her that we don't need to talk about our business in front of other people. People think she is hilarious, but it's not funny to me. The other night we partied until about 3 am. I had way too much to drink. My wife wanted to have sex when we got home, but I was too intoxicated to get an erection. Didn't she tell my partners the next day? She kept referring to me as limp dick. I think that arguing around other people gives her confidence, but she wouldn't like it if I treated her this way."

87. Pretending to be helpless.

"My girlfriend wants me to gas up her car, take out her garbage and carry every package for her, even if it's a stick of gum. I know that some people may think I am not being a gentleman, but I don't like it when a woman expects me to do things for her that she can do for herself. What if I expected her to wash my clothes and cook my dinner everyday, just because she is a woman. I don't mind putting together bookshelves, helping her carry bags or even opening her car door. But you know, God help those who help themselves. When I see a woman who is independent and strong, it's something about her that makes me want to help her even more."

88. Not being spontaneous and flexible with the sexual relationship.

"My wife and I moved to our new house a few years ago. The kids were with her parents. We had spent the entire day moving into our new home. I will never forget, that day my wife was wearing these tight, lime-green stretch pants and a see-through t-shirt. Her hair was tousled from sweating and moving boxes. She looked so sexy to me. When we finished moving the things into the house, I begged her to make love to me right there on the living room floor. She refused to do it. She told me that she was sweaty and dirty and she didn't feel comfortable having sex. She also said that she didn't think that we should be thinking about having sex with boxes strewn about the living room floor. My wife cannot function sexually unless she is freshly showered, in the bed, with the lights off. Sometimes, I want to smell her natural body odor. I want to take off her panty hose and kiss off her lipstick. The dishes don't need to be washed, and clothes folded, before we make love. I enjoyed our relationship so much more when we were just dating."

89. Testing the relationship by making him jealous.

"Every guy on my girlfriend's job has a crush on her and wants to marry her, according to her. She tells me this all the time, to make me jealous. Check this out, she even sent herself flowers, but told me they were from a secret admirer. I found the receipt on her credit card. Now isn't that pathetic? I feel like, if I got to fight for a woman's heart, I don't want it. I am not going to compete for somebody's love. This type of game playing does not make me want to marry her—or jealous. It just makes me think that she is dishonest and a game player."

90. Not compromising on social activities.

"My wife's company's functions are mandatory events that will compromise the relationship if I don't attend. Little get-togethers at my friend's home and my family cabarets are ghetto affairs and a waste of her precious time. Does she really think that I have a good time with her stuck-up, phony co-workers? No! I go because I love and respect her. I didn't go to the last to functions her job sponsored because she didn't go to my parent's 50th wedding anniversary dinner. She claimed that she was sick, but when I called home was not in. Came to find out later that week that she went to a show with her sister and two of her friends. I still love her, but I feel like our worlds don't mix. I am at the point now where, if she can't compromise and do some of the things that are important to me, I can tell you point blank, I know that this marriage is not going to last."

91. Not admitting when she is wrong.

"You're wasting your time writing a book about what women do wrong. You know women don't ever think that they do anything wrong. Anything that they do that might be wrong, a man made them do it and deserved it. I married my wife because she is the only woman who has ever admitted to me that she was wrong. I think it's so sexy for a woman to have the courage to be accountable for her own behavior. I knew my wife and I would make it through thick and thin, because she is the type of person who is willing to learn from her mistakes. I was right—we've been married over 36 years."

92. Calling him when he is out with his friends to curse him out or to tell him that he is homeless.

"I feel trapped in my marriage. What the heck was I thinking when I decided to marry this woman. It's simple—if I am not at work when she calls, I am cheating. My wife loves to call me whenever I am out with the boys to say, 'I hope they have an extra bed, because you can't sleep here tonight.' Why can't I go out with my friends to play cards or listen to a jazz band? I always ask her to go, but she refuses. I am sick and tired of being kicked out of my own home for no reason. One of these nights I am never going to come home again."

93. Holding a grudge after they have come to an accord.

"One night on a whim, my friends and I went to Chicago. It was totally unplanned; we were gone for three days. I called my fiancé to let her know what was going on. She was devastated. She accused me of not loving her and not caring about her feelings. I told her that I was very sorry and that it was an irresponsible thing for me to do. I begged and pleaded with her to forgive me. We made up, so I thought, but it's been three months and she still barely speaks to me. I don't want to lose her because she is the best thing that has ever happened to me. But the stress of being in a relationship with someone who holds a grudge is unbearable. When I know that I love a person and want to be with them, once we both understand each other's position, I am ready to move on. To me life is too short to hold grudges. One day you're going to look back on your life and think about all the stupid time that you spent angry that you could have spent making love."

94. Acting ashamed of him in front of her friends.

"I couldn't believe that I allowed my self to date a woman who admitted to me that she was ashamed of me while in college. She said that all of her friend's boyfriends drove expensive sports cars. I drove a rusted out Nova. She never invited me to any of her sorority parties. I never met her family. But I was good enough to buy her textbooks for two semesters and gave her money every week for food and personal items. The sex was amazing, and to be frank, I couldn't believe a girl that was so good looking would give me the time of day. One day I saw her on campus and I walked up behind her and kissed her on her neck. She froze turned around and called me a creep. That's been 20 years ago and it still hurts to this day. No self-respecting human being should spend time with a person who is ashamed of them. When I think back on this event, I am not angry with her, I am angry with me for thinking so little of myself."

95. Ripping apart his self-esteem by telling him that he is like his "no good daddy."

"I have always had a complex about my father leaving me when I was a teenager. My mother would get angry with me and tell me that I was good for nothing just like my daddy. I felt like some one was stabbing me in my soul. But you know, boys are not supposed to cry, so I would pretend that it didn't bother me. My father cheated on my mother and every one in the neighborhood knew this. He was also an alcoholic and he beat my mother when he drank too much. I am embarrassed to say this, but I still loved my daddy. He taught me how to catch a ball, we went fishing together and he helped me with my school homework. My dad had a great sense of humor and he always told me that he loved me in spite of the marital problems with my mother. Regardless of his mistakes, flaws and imperfections, he is still the man whose blood runs through my veins, and I shouldn't have to feel ashamed of loving my father. My high school girl friend told me that I was no good, like my daddy, and it took everything inside of me not to hit her. That was the last time I talked to her. Now I am reluctant to talk, to women I date, about my father. They think that the reason that I won't discuss my father is because I hate him, but this is not true. It's because I love him. Father and son relationships are touchy topics for most men. I would tell a woman that if a man opens up to you about his truest feelings for his father, she has been trusted with his heart. If she uses this information to tear him down, even in a heated argument, she could lose him forever."

96. Acting phony when she's around other people.

"The way my wife talks, laughs and acts around other people sickens me to my stomach. She uses this high-pitched phony voice that is disgusting. Why can't she just be herself? No, I take it back, I don't know which person is the real her. When no one is looking, she is much funnier and down-to-earth. She thinks that she impresses other people, but they actually talk about her behind her back. They think that she is phony and fake. I'll never tell her, but even my family think that she acts fake. To me, there is nothing sexier than a person confident enough to be themselves, no matter who is around."

97. Not making him a priority in her life.

"My girlfriend is working on her master's degree and she has a full and part-time job. I love the fact that she is ambitious and hard working, but I rarely get a chance to see her. Usually, when we spend time together, she is grouchy, sleepy, tired and no fun to be around. I tell her that she gives me the leftover crumbs of who she is. It's been two months or more since we had sex. She tells me that she wants to settle down and have children one day. I would like to spend some time with her to determine if we are even compatible. If she can't invest in the relationship now, I don't see how a marriage would have any priority in her life. I haven't told her yet, but I am planning to see someone else. I am looking forward to developing a relationship with someone who has time to go out and enjoy life more. By the time my girlfriend even realizes that I am gone, I'll probably be married with three children."

98. Taking advice from friends and relatives about how to conduct the relationship.

"I can't imagine asking my family or friends for their opinion on whether or not I should leave the woman I love; or telling them the personal, intimate details of our relationship. Women are supposed to be so much smarter than men when it comes to relationships and feelings, but I don't think this is true. I feel that women are more inclined to ask for advice from their girlfriends, mommas and sisters, oh yeah and Cosmopolitan, on what to do in a relationship rather than follow their own hearts. How can somebody, who has only a one sided view of who I am, give her an honest opinion about our relationship? Hell, they don't know me! They only know what she tells them about me. I bet she doesn't tell the foul things that she does to hurt the relationship. And the crazy thing is, most of the women that they ask for relationship advice, don't even have a man and have never been in a healthy relationship. 'Girl you better leave him, he ain't no good' that's all their man-less girlfriends tell them. But if I gave just one of them the time of day, they would stab her in the back and jump in the sack with me, before she could blink her eyes. I was crazy about this girl. We broke up over some he-says-she-says boloney. When I date a girl and I find out her decisions are not coming from her heart, I don't need her."

99. Wanting him to guess what is bothering her.

"I hate when a woman tells me that everything is fine, but her behavior indicates otherwise. I keep asking her 'baby what's wrong.' She says, 'nothing,' while at the same time rolling her eyes with these weird facial expressions. I ask her, 'baby is everything okay?' She says, 'yes,' but at the same time she is sleeping on the couch and giving me the silent treatment. I am not a mind reader. If something is bothering a woman she should be mature enough to tell me what is really bothering her, not treat me like dirt and hope that we figure it out."

100. Not using extra care to upkeep her hygiene when she is on her period.

"I had five sisters and I could never tell when they were on their periods. My mother was very strict about hygiene and keeping the house clean. I don't know how other men feel about this but I am disgusted when I go in the bathroom and a woman leaves a pad or tampon unwrapped in the trash can; or when she leaves her soiled panties on the bedroom floor. I think more women need to have dignity about being a woman. I know this is a different, topic but I feel the same way when I see a pregnant woman with tight clothing over her stomach. Whatever happened to modesty and taking some type of pride in the process of motherhood? I still like a woman who closes the door when she uses the bathroom, and displays some type of privacy and decency about herself."

101. Blaming him for her problems.

"It's not my fault that she hates her job. It's not my fault that she dropped out of college. It's not my fault that she lives beyond her means and cannot afford to pay her rent. I am not her sugar daddy or her savior. Women don't understand the pressure they put men under to make their lives run smoothly. I dated this girl in law school. We were both struggling financially, working three jobs, and pulling all night study sessions. She took me home to meet her parents during the Christmas break. I couldn't believe that her mother told her, 'You can do better for yourself. If you have to struggle while dating him, you don't need him. You need a man who can help you, child.' My girlfriend, at the time, was humiliated. I asked her if she felt that her mom was right, she said 'no.' Six months later our relationship was over and she was dating a married accountant 20 years her senior. She moved to a condo uptown and started wearing expensive clothes and bought a new car. I think as much as women deny it, deep inside they think men are responsible for what is wrong in their life. This is why I am now looking for a woman with herself together. I don't want to be somebody's hero, I want somebody to love me unconditionally."

102. Selling your self cheap but want me to pay for what you're giving away to other guys for free.

I worked with a woman in the factory who was very promiscuous. Many of the guys in my work crew had had sex with her. She was no beauty, but she had a big a—. As a matter of fact, she had a reputation of having good stuff. I could tell that she had a crush on me. Sometimes she would make lunch for me or ask me out to dinner. I decided to take her up on her offer for dinner one evening at her home. After dinner, I tried to entice her into having sex with me, but she adamantly refused. She suggested that we hold each other, have breakfast in the morning and catch an early afternoon movie. I was confused because several of the fellows on my job had sex with her in their cars and hotels. These guys are not the kind of guys to lie about sleeping with a woman. This was not high school. I told her that I was not interested in a long term relationship, but felt that we had sexual chemistry and that she wanted me as much as I wanted to her. She agreed, but said that because she wanted a "real-relationship" with me, she didn't want to ruin her chances by having sex too early. Can you believe this! Here she is giving it away for free to every guy who ask, now she wants me to pay for it by wining and dining her. Hell no! What turns me off is a woman who wants me to treat her like a queen, yet she acts like a tramp.

103. Putting my sexual desires over the emotional needs of her children.

I dated a woman who told her crying toddler that she could not sleep in her bed that night because she was sleeping with me. We had been dating around 6 months, but I lost all respect for this woman after this incident. I never called her again. How could any woman, let a man that she is dating take precedence over her child? I would never kick my child out of the bed to sleep with some woman that I am dating. My two boys come first in my life. Any guy, who is worth a hill of beans, would never want a woman to put his emotional needs before the emotional needs of her children.

978-0-595-46589-7
0-595-46589-7